The Solution Group

Positive Change through the Group Process

by
Bruce C. Dawson

New View Publications
Chapel Hill

*This book is for Diane Gossen, who, in simple terms,
just told me to go ahead,
and to Betty, who is with me for a wonderful life.*

The Solution Group. Copyright © 1993 by Bruce Dawson

Library of Congress Cataloging-in-Publication Data
Dawson, Bruce C., 1947-
      The solution group: positive change through the group
      process
      1. Substance abuse—Treatment   2. Group psychotherapy
      3. Reality therapy   4. Control theory
I. Title
RC564.F38 1993   616.86'0651--dc20   93-8758
ISBN 0-944337-16-3

ACKNOWLEDGMENTS

I am indebted to William Glasser, M.D., whose reality therapy and control theory provided me the theoretical framework for understanding what I had learned "by the seat of my pants" in my personal life and in my professional experience as an addictions counselor.

I have learned and borrowed much from my reality therapist colleagues to whom I am ever grateful. The Thinking/Feeling activity in Chapter 5 is based on an exercise done by Diane Gossen in my first intensive week of training in reality therapy. Diane Gossen, who continues to encourage me, is also responsible for the analysis of the "control car" presented in Chapter 7, and the relationship maps described in Chapter 8. Perry Good developed the basic needs circle used in Chapter 9. Perry's publisher/husband Fred and her editor/friend Nancy Salmon are largely responsible for transforming my ideas into coherent words so they may be shared with friends, colleagues, and others who want to help people make important changes in their lives. Thanks also to Angela Whitlock-Dove, in-house editor for this book.

And finally, many thanks to Barnes Boffey for the Quality World challenge he presented to me, and to Linda Geronilla for her continued support.

INTRODUCTION

When given a choice between doing individual or group therapy, most therapists would choose individual therapy. Why?

First, the logistics of individual therapy are less complicated; it takes more energy to schedule a group of people. There are also other issues such as: Who should be put in a group? How do you get all the people to start at the same time? What do you do for follow-up?

Second, therapists are sometimes intimidated by the idea of doing group therapy because they do not feel qualified to run groups. Group therapy is considered to be more complicated and sophisticated than individual therapy because it requires advanced levels of knowledge and training. With this book, Bruce Dawson has simplified the group process by making his Solution Groups easy to initiate and less threatening to operate.

There were numerous things that initially attracted me to the Solution Group. The groups could be run with any age clients—adolescents and adults can work together to find solutions. The group could be operated in either a closed or open-ended fashion, with clients being added after the starting date. Finally, the planned sequence of discussion topics are presented in a very simple, non-threatening manner which helps clients relax and have fun while learning.

After hearing Bruce present at the 1992 International Reality Therapy Convention in Vancouver, I invited him to train my therapy staff in the Solution Group process. Since then we have been doing Solution Groups with great success—attendance and participation have been outstanding. Even our counselors now make positive comments like, "I learned a great deal myself by running the group."

I express my gratitude to Bruce Dawson for having created a practical way for both client and therapist to have fun learning reality therapy together in their journey to create solutions and live more responsibly.

Linda S. Geronilla, Ph. D.
Director, Associates in Counseling and Training, Inc.
Charleston, West Virginia

TABLE OF CONTENTS

UNDERLYING CONCEPTS

I was skeptical at first. I suspected that what I had learned in my first intensive week of training in reality therapy might just be so much bologna, so I decided to test it out. I cannot recall who my first victim was, but I remember asking the questions: "So if that's how you're feeling, what are you thinking? What are you doing? How is that working out for you?" Much to my amazement, I immediately saw some positive results. I used what I learned from that first experience with my next client, and from that experience with the next. My knowledge grew. When I applied what I had learned in that first week of reality therapy training, my clients gained ground in their recovery.

In addition to doing individual counseling, I was also conducting several hours of group sessions every day. My training had focused exclusively on using reality therapy in one-on-one counseling situations, but I saw no reason why the same approach couldn't benefit clients in group sessions as well. I visualized the reality therapy process allowing my clients to grow without subjecting them to attack or the diminishing activities commonly used in groups. With additional instruction in reality therapy and control theory, encouragement from the people who trained me, trial and error and close attention to what my clients told me, I gradually developed the process I call "The Solution Group." Its effectiveness does not depend on the specific participants nor on their specific problems. I have trained others to conduct Solution Groups and they have experienced similar success. In the safe, non-coercive environment of the Solution Group, clients make effective and meaningful changes in their lives, and all steps leading to these changes are accomplished in a positive, relaxed atmosphere.

The Solution Group process is grounded in control theory and reality therapy as developed by William Glasser, MD. Control theory, first articulated by William Powers, provides a way to explain our behavior; reality therapy helps people to change their behavior when they want to do so. The participants in a Solution Group are continuously being educated about control theory and reality therapy, although not in a pedantic way. I never say, "Today we are going to learn about control theory!" The participants don't want to learn a theory; they want something that works. My strategy is to have them understand the concepts and use them effectively before I tell them what it is they are learning and where they can go to learn more. The control theory/reality therapy approach thus comes to have true meaning to them as something that is practical, not just theoretical.

Because of their fundamental importance, I want to present briefly some of the basic concepts of control theory and reality therapy, as I interpret them, before embarking on a description of the logistics and procedures involved in conducting the Solution Group. Experienced reality therapists may want to skim through the rest of this chapter or jump ahead to the next. If you are being introduced to control theory and reality therapy for the first time, however, I encourage you to supplement my cursory explanations with some more comprehensive presentations of these subjects (see Appendix).

Control theory explains the "why" and "how" of what we're doing all the time, which is behaving. I used to view only my physical actions as behavior, but with knowledge of control theory came a different perspective, that of total behavior. The control theory idea of total behavior, simply stated, is that our thoughts, actions, feelings, and physiology are all parts of our total behavior, and these elements are inextricably linked. Therefore, what we think affects what we do, how we feel, and our health. Our feelings and health carry with them equally powerful consequences for our thoughts and actions.

During my younger days I experienced a period of terrible loneliness. I spent many sleepless nights in my apartment, all alone, trying to figure out how to stop feeling lonely. All the elements of total behavior were there, operating together: thinking (no one loves me), feeling (lonely, unhappy), actions (staying in my apartment), and physiology (sleeplessness). Looking back at this period of my life, after learning something about control theory and reality therapy, I understood that by thinking no one loved me and by staying in the apartment all through those sleepless nights, of course I was going to be lonely! How could there be any other outcome? The key to overcoming my loneliness was changing those parts of my total behavior over which I had the most control—doing and thinking. Once I started to go out and do things with other people and thought that it was possible to make friends, I began to feel better about myself and be happier. I no longer lay awake at night. As parts of my total behavior changed, the other parts changed with them!

Dr. Glasser has provided a model of total behavior in comparing human behavior to a car with front-wheel drive. Action, thinking, feeling, and physiology are each represented by one of the car's four wheels. The most powerful parts of total behavior, action and thinking, are the front wheels, where the car's power and steering originate. Nothing on a car acts completely independently. A decision to drive at high speed and turn left affects more than just the two front wheels. As the accelerator descends and the steering wheel turns, the entire car careens around a curve at high speed, proof that the whole car's "behavior" is linked to the behavior of the front wheels. The same rule applies to human actions, thoughts, feelings, and physiology. What we think and do directly affects our feelings and our physical health.

Dr. Glasser's control theory states that we are all internally driven to meet certain needs, which he identifies as love, power, freedom, fun, and survival. Some people refer to the need for love as "belonging" and the need for power as "achievement" or "recognition." The acronym I use to help my groups remember these critical needs is "L.A.F.F.S."—Love, Achievement, Freedom, Fun, and Survival. Control theory maintains that when any of our needs is threatened or not being met, we *must* do something. This is one thing that we have no choice about. Many times we may not consciously recognize that a need is unmet, and sometimes our behavior may not seem sensible to other people, or even to ourselves. I myself occasionally wonder why at times I feel afraid when to my thinking there is nothing to be afraid of. In fact, thinking is only a part of my total behavior. The entire system—including thinking, doing, feeling, and physiology—is greater than any one part, and if that system, at any level, perceives a need that is not being met, then the system will behave to meet that particular need. In spite of every intention that we may have to do nothing in a given situation, we will do something anyway. Even if we only panic or think, we are still doing something. The variety of behaviors we might engage in is nearly inexhaustible. During group sessions my clients usually come up with no less than six dozen behaviors that they get into when they perceive their needs being threatened. The question is not whether we are or are not behaving, but whether the behaviors that we adopt are helping us to get what we really want.

This brings me to the reality therapy part of this discussion. In the case of my loneliness, the recovery process was breaking down for me at the evaluation level. The various routes to a solution that I tried were not working out. I was focusing on what I did not have instead of what I wanted, and I couldn't see that what I was doing was not getting me what I wanted. Funny as it seems, the most important question, "Is what I am doing getting me what I want?", had not been asked. When it finally was asked, I changed my behavior. Evaluation questions are the heart of the reality therapy process. Any question that leads to change can be a part of the process, but open-ended questions are most productive. "Are you happy?" is a closed-ended question. "If you were happy, what would that mean to you?" is an open-ended question. Obviously, the second question opens up a wider range of possibilities. Instead of asking questions that can be answered with yes or no, it is better to ask questions that call for more information and lead the clients towards their stated goals.

During the group process, the clients are asked to evaluate all their behaviors on how they are working out for them, not on whether the behaviors are wrong or right. This is extremely important! The evaluation should always be based on how effective the behavior is. I never ask the participants whether something is right or wrong, or good or bad. The safe environment of the group is carefully created by this line of evaluation. My clients have never done very well in a "right or wrong" world. I do not question them on that basis.

Some of the evaluation questions that could be asked are: How is this behavior working out? Is this behavior going to help you get what you want? If you weren't doing this, what would you be doing? If you were happy, what would you be doing? The essential element of this type of questioning is the implication that the clients have choices. When the clients come into the group they are often unaware that they have choices, yet they are constantly making choices every day, even if they do not like the choices that they have. The educational part of my job is to help them see this. The rest of my job entails having them evaluate how their choices are working out for them, and helping them find other choices they can make to get what they want.

The part of control theory that deals with "real wants" is referred to as the "quality world." In our quality worlds we store the mental pictures of things we want, things that we believe will satisfy our needs. One of my clients, Janet, tells the group that she is lonely and wants to find someone who understands her. Is it her needs or wants that are driving her behavior? How do a client's wants relate to needs? Our wants are the way we translate our needs. When we are in pain and our thinking is confused, our expressed wants may not be an accurate translation of our needs, but they are valid indicators nonetheless. After further talking, Janet sees that her need for love and belonging isn't being met. Identifying and finding an alternative, healthy way to fulfill that need could satisfy Janet more than a never-ending search for that elusive "someone who understands."

During introductions with a new group, I find out from the participants what they really want. It always seems to come down to happiness, peace, or some variation on that theme, even though they might set conditions on what that would look like to them. Once the wants of the group members have been clarified, whatever their individual circumstances and problems happen to be, the clients recognize a common bond in wanting the same thing. We then spend time talking about what that world of happiness or peace might look like. The entire process helps the participants develop their quality picture of what life will look like when (not *if*) they get what they want—what they really want!

While clients consistently and freely evaluate how their current actions are working out and how they might work if continued into the future, a much more unfamiliar task for them is coming up with new behaviors to replace the old ones that haven't been working. (Notice I am not using the word *difficult*—the task is just unfamiliar.) To help clients develop their ability to find alternative behaviors, I constantly direct them to evaluate their own lives and current behaviors. In fact, asking evaluative questions has become habitual, whether or not I am leading a group.

Unlike many groups where topics of discussion arise by happenstance, in the Solution Group there is a planned sequence of discussion topics and activities. Members of the Solution Group are given the chores of exploring their total behavior, evaluating their lives, discovering their needs, and beginning the process of making new choices. One of the greatest benefits of using control theory and reality therapy in groups is that group members learn from each other. When they receive individual counseling, clients are limited to learning from themselves and, perhaps, the counselor. In the group, the evaluative questions that apply to themselves apply to others as well, so they are collectively evaluating as the process evolves. The counselor consistently asks evaluative questions while educating the group about control theory/reality therapy concepts. Clients, in general, are looking for direction; however, they do not need nor are they looking for someone to tell them what to do. It pleases me greatly when a client makes a dramatic turnaround, yet cannot think of one thing that I ever told him to do! Letting the clients do the work is of paramount importance. The remainder of this book describes the process I have developed using Dr. Glasser's control theory and reality therapy to direct the group participants in their "solutions."

STRATEGIES AND STRUCTURE

STRATEGIES

The Solution Group attends to the wants and needs of each group member in a positive, non-critical environment. At the same time that there is identification through the peer process (always a benefit of group work), the Solution Group consistently focuses on the individual, which is one thing that distinguishes this process from a standard group. Each and every person who enters the Solution Group is promised a lot. They are promised a safe environment, free from criticism or judgment on the basis of past behavior. They are promised an environment where their life is evaluated on *how it is working out for them,* not on whether it is good or bad, and not on whether it is right or wrong. They have the chance to continue to self-evaluate as each of the other members talks. In the end their group "bonding" is very intense, based on the attraction of everybody really wanting to have the same things (happiness, peace)—not their wanting to get rid of the same things (fear or guilt, for instance). As one participant remarked, "This group did not get me to attack my thinking. It gave me a chance to change my beliefs about myself."

Two of the challenges I had when starting out were how to get full attendance at every group meeting and how to get everyone to be a cooperative, willing participant. As a former salesman I already knew the answer—give them what they want! So every day ends on a positive focus. What do you want? How can you get it? We end each day planning solutions. The Solution Group never dwells on how difficult it has been coping with particular feelings, thoughts, or actions. Instead we work towards solutions for these destructive feelings and the challenges they bring. We talk of what it would be like if the clients were doing, thinking, and feeling what they wanted. This positive focus is maintained throughout the entire group process. Discussion centers on the areas in their lives where the clients, individually and as a group, declare that they are having their greatest challenges. This contributes to success because it means we go first to the areas that, in the clients' minds, have primary importance. We do not remain focused on what initiated the crises in their lives; we simply discuss the outcomes in terms of behavior. The benefit here is that the clients can come up with other behaviors that do not have the same painful outcomes, but will still help them get what they want.

Evaluative questions seem to unify the group. As one client after another is asked these questions— "How's it working out for you?" "Do you want to make a change in how it's been working out?"—they begin to realize that they are all in the same boat. Every person in the group wants a change and this is a unifying force. It surprises them to find that other people want the same things they want and that it's okay.

Perhaps the most important aspect of the process is that it is non-threatening and non-critical. Each client is asked to participate, and the group moves no faster than the slowest member. Participants are not criticized for being unable to detect or clarify their feelings. As a matter of fact, many people who are emotionally distraught do not know how to describe what they are feeling or thinking. But the questions are asked several times, in several different ways, and it helps them to hear what the others say.

Surprisingly, denial is not an issue in the Solution Group. When the Solution Group process is being followed, denial evaporates! Criminal, addictive, violent, and abusive behaviors, along with resulting thoughts and feelings, are openly and willingly admitted. The process seems to open a door the client can choose to step through, not be forced through by threats or fear of punishment.

There is no berating of group members for any past behaviors, no negative feedback. Group members do not criticize each other; the emphasis is on *self*-evaluation, not evaluating anybody else. Disclosures that help lead to a recovery solution are met with the appropriate, respectful feedback. This is an opportunity for the client to find ways of doing something differently the next time.

Many professionals believe they achieve the best results by psychologically beating up their clients, reducing them to a compliant shell. As I see it, the client already knows what he/she has been doing; the Solution Group allows him/her the dignity to discover the truth without suffering abuse. That doesn't mean, however, that honesty is abandoned in favor of kindness. Clients appreciate the frankness and honesty of a counselor who is always open and asking sincere questions.

CLIENTS

Most of the clients in my groups are referred to me by other services, other counselors, ex-clients, or friends. They come from all walks of life. Many counselors feel that six to eight clients makes an ideal group, but I am most comfortable with groups of eight to twelve. Even larger groups are fine. Solution Group activities work best when input from the clients is extensive and varied, so it helps to have many people participating. The mix of backgrounds, experiences, and problems among the clients in a group can vary dramatically. One group that I recently worked with included professionals, convicts, addicts, and non-addicts. After years of refining the Solution Group process, I am convinced that it is equally effective with in-patient and out-patient groups. Initially I doubted that out-patients would benefit from each other's experience or bond very well. Not true!

All clients should be approached with the expectation that they have the potential to succeed. In their own minds they think this is probably impossible, so they don't need a counselor affirming their doomsday thinking. Try not to approach your clients as the sum of their past drinking, violence, or any other form of misbehavior. Look at them simply as "behaving" people, not as bad or misbehaving people.

I make an effort to like my clients. Whenever this is a struggle, and it can be, using control theory and reality therapy helps. Here is an example. Ted, referred to my group from the correctional system, was extremely antagonistic. Never having had a close home life, he had been living on his own since he was fourteen. Now in his early twenties, Ted acted like a belligerent adolescent. In group he was disruptive and uncooperative. He stated clearly that he was unwilling to trust anyone. During his first week he also stated that he did not perceive that his needs were being met by anyone in his personal life or in the correctional system. Ted's options were limited. Leaving the group meant returning to jail. Although he said he wanted help, he did nothing in group to convince me or the others that he really meant it. After a week, we talked privately. Not wanting to go back to jail, Ted stated that he wanted to complete the group process that we had started. He agreed that if he was going to complete the program he might as well get something he wanted out of it. We agreed that he would make a list of four or five things he wanted. He returned with a list of over twenty surprisingly varied items. We selected one to work on first. Once I knew what Ted wanted—to let people know that he could care for them—not only did he start to make progress, but he magically became more likable.

To get results like this the counselor has to get involved with the clients. Many professionals expound the virtues of mental, emotional, and physical distance between themselves and their clients. They avoid walking through patient lounges and never mingle with clients outside of group meetings. While this keeps a counselor "protected" from the client, it also "protects" the counselor from an opportunity. In coffee lounges, for instance, where clients are relaxed and humor occurs naturally, casual encounters begin the process of humanizing the counselor. It is important, of course, that you are seen first and foremost in your true role as a counselor, but clients want to know everything there is to know about success, and it is important to them to know what success looks like on a regular, familiar basis. People who are looking for a way to change their lives are intensely interested in anyone they know who has done it. One of the keys to success in Twelve-Step programs is the tradition of "attraction, rather than promotion." When I mingle and occasionally have coffee with my clients, I know that I appear more trustworthy and approachable. Still, the time I spend with them is random and they respect my need to mix with co-workers too. I simply try to treat my clients as I would other people. A final comment regarding this issue: I do not invite my clients home. But, if they want to know what I did to resolve issues in my life, I tell them. If they want to know if I think I've been successful, I tell them.

Many of the clients and situations discussed in this book have been compiled from my years of experience as an addictions counselor. I frequently use addicted clients as examples because I have worked with so many of them, and they are notorious for being difficult. Furthermore, no addicted client is free from other issues that need attention: bulimia, anorexia, sexual abuse, violence (giver and receiver), criminal behavior, and so on. This doesn't mean, however, that the success of using control theory/reality therapy in the Solution Group is limited to clients struggling to overcome alcohol or drug abuse, to name two of the more common addictions. I have also worked with youth groups and business groups, in-patients and out-patients, in all sorts of group settings. The process is effective for all.

Let me now introduce you to the members of a typical group, clients I will be using as examples in the following chapters. These are not real people, but composites of many clients I have worked with in the past.

Janet - age 21. Bulimic. Addicted to drugs. Recently released from hospitalization for attempted suicide. Single mother. College drop-out. States she hates the world. Doesn't see any relationships in her life that are of any value.

George - age 42. Alcoholic. Has been through three marriages. Feels and thinks that he is a total failure. Wants proof for everything.

Ted - age 22. Drug addict. Referred by legal system. Must complete counseling to stay out of jail. Has been in and out of jail since age 14. Father was violent and abusive alcoholic. Sees mother and self as victims. States that he trusts no one.

Laurel - age 38. Battered wife. Co-dependent. Living with active alcoholic who physically abuses her and her children. Laurel constantly uses excuses to make it okay for this to happen.

Robert - age 17. Rebellious. Expelled from school due to skipping classes. His parents claim he has a "typical" teenage attitude. Not happy to be here. Complying with everyone else to take pressure off.

Anita - age 26. Physically abused. Portrays self as victim, always depressed and suffering. "Everything would be all right if everyone else would..." Chronic worrier. Sexually abused from age 8-14.

Albert - age 32. States openly that he is going to commit suicide. A native American, he is not happy to be working with white people, but doesn't want to go to native resources. Doesn't talk much; looks at floor primarily. Very apologetic. Sexually abused as youth.

Marge - age 38. Says she is not able to form any meaningful relationships. Has had several disastrous affairs. Can't get along with anyone in her family, especially her mother. Professional.

Charles - age 50. Unhappy. Describes himself as being depressed. The manager of a large business. Says he has everything he ever wanted, but does not feel connected to anyone, including family.

GUIDELINES

There are only two strict guidelines in the group: confidentiality and prohibition of alcohol and other drugs. The most important aspect of these guidelines is that if they are breached the result should be a consequence rather than a punishment. Almost every client knows a lot about punishment. They all know how they have been punished by others, and they are pros at punishing themselves. One must beware, however, that what one person considers a consequence could well be viewed as punishment to the person receiving it. What may be a natural consequence to the group facilitator may be perceived as total rejection by the client. The rule I follow in the Solution Group is that the clients name their own consequences and then enact them. This way the clients become responsible for their own behavior. Although strict guidelines do exist, I myself have never had to impose any kind of consequence on a group member. My job is to ensure that they learn about true consequences and that they are not too hard on themselves. A turning point in recovery can be the moment when a person grasps the concept of consequences. Once, a client decided on his own to check into a detox center, then later he returned to complete treatment successfully. By witnessing the success of a consequential approach firsthand, everyone else in the whole group benefited.

Historically, alcohol and drug treatment centers have thrown people out if they have used prohibited substances during the course of treatment. What purpose is such punishment supposed to serve? Promising to expel someone is not a solution-oriented consequence. Finding assistance for a client to withdraw from drugs or alcohol and then bring them back into the group is. It helps all concerned to know that they will not be summarily expelled for what is, after all, expected activity for an addict—substance abuse. Instead, we work to find an individual plan that will help the client learn from his or her own behavior. Effective results come once the client is able to determine his or her own fate.

There are also several less official guidelines that the group follows. We observe a no-smoking policy, so we try to have a short break every 45 minutes or so. Some time is devoted each day to hellos and closure. Everyone is urged to sit in a different chair at each group meeting. In my own experience during recovery I liked to find "a home away from home," a secure spot where I could recede into my own little world. It is gratifying to hear a group enforcing the changing of seats after a few days, mutually helping each other find a new spot. Guidelines shouldn't, however, take precedence over an individual client's needs. Anita, for instance, disturbed by prior experiences of rape and violence, insisted at the first meeting that she must always sit next to the door. Remembering that changing seats is only a guideline, I was able to get Anita to agree to move to another chair when she thought and felt she was safe. How long did that take? Only three days! Because the group respected the guideline and policed their own seating arrangements, they noticed when Anita changed her behavior. As Anita successfully changed seats for the next few days, much ado was made and congratulations offered, reminding her of her triumph.

At each step of the way, every group member is asked for their input. I usually ask, "Who wants to go next?" When no one answers, I interrupt the silence with, "Oops, perhaps I should have asked who *will* go next?" This invariably produces chuckles, and most of the time, someone then agrees. If there is still no volunteer, I pick on someone, gently reassuring them that "everyone will have a turn eventually, so you might as well go now as later."

Perhaps the most important guideline, mentioned before, is not to move any faster than the slowest member of the group. I check frequently for understanding by asking, "Does that make sense?" or "Do you understand what I'm saying?" If someone does not understand, we stop until that person is able to comprehend. Sometimes a reluctant member is bypassed at the beginning of a discussion, but drawn in again later, thus validating the importance of their contribution. There is nothing in this group process that is so important that it has to be done by a particular time. The program is for the clients, so it has to proceed at their speed, not the counselor's. I do, however, make a point of ending group meetings on time every day. The clients soon learn that solutions don't arrive any faster by running overtime. They can actually find solutions outside of group as well, which is one of the nicest outcomes of all. The clients, though strangers at first, quickly begin working with each other. They start driving each other to appointments and supporting the need each has to recover.

The most important skills a counselor needs are questioning, listening, paraphrasing, summarizing, and remembering. If you don't have a good memory, keep notes! The success of the model depends on practice, practice, and more practice. Don't be afraid to tailor the model to suit your own needs and setting. One-hour group sessions are not ideal, but if that is all the time you have, go for it!

The Solution Group process takes all participants through the various aspects of their lives, encouraging them to evaluate for themselves how their behaviors have been working out for them. The stages of the process are as follows:

1. Introductions
2. Feelings
3. Thinking
4. Actions
5. Physiology and Total Behavior
6. How Relationships Are Affected by Behavior
7. How Relationships Meet One's Needs
8. WIN/WIN Solutions
9. Good-byes and Follow-Up

This sequence has proven to be the most effective for me. There is no strict schedule, and the stages do not necessarily correspond to specific group meetings in a series. The group moves along only as fast as the slowest member, so work on any stage overflows to the next meeting if we haven't covered everything we need to when time runs out. The important thing is that we never end a session on a sour note. I named this process the "Solution Group" because that characterizes its ultimate aim as well as its daily format.

INTRODUCTIONS
Stage One

KEY QUESTIONS
What has been going on that led to your coming to group?
What have you done to try to resolve your problems?
How did it work out? Did it help you get what you want?
What do you want?
If you got that, what would it mean to you?

ACTIVITIES
Questioning of individual clients to elicit information about what they want and to begin evaluations of what they have been doing.

From the clients' point of view, during introductions they become acquainted with each other as well as with what is going to be happening during the group process. My intention during the introductions, on the other hand, is to gather information about the clients that I will need to conduct the group for the remainder of the sessions—that is, what the clients think they want, what they really want, and what they have tried doing to get what they want. At the same time, I begin right away to prod the clients to evaluate the effectiveness of their own behaviors.

In the introductory session, all members of the group are asked, one at a time, to tell their names, where they are from, a little bit about themselves, what brought them to group, and finally what results they want from the group. By asking a lot of questions during the introductory process, I begin the process of having each of the clients self-evaluate. The specific focus of the Solution Group is not what the clients might have done in their past nor whether it was good or bad, right or wrong, but rather how they perceive the effectiveness of their past behaviors. George, for instance, can evaluate whether his drinking behavior has been getting him what he wants even while denying that he is an "alcoholic." After everyone in the group has been introduced, I introduce myself, briefly describing my own background. By disclosing my own personal history, I build a connection with the group so that they perceive me not as someone above and apart from the group, but as someone like themselves. The subtle message is that if I could figure out how to overcome my difficulties, they can learn how to overcome theirs. At the end of this stage I outline the rules and guidelines that the group will be following in the remaining sessions. Perhaps the best way to help you to understand how I conduct the introductory process is to demonstrate with a couple of examples. We'll start with Charles.

Charles gives his name and states that he is from a nearby town where he grew up. He has not done much traveling, but on vacation he likes to go to Hawaii. He goes on to state that he has never been in a group setting before and doesn't really know what else to say. I ask him what had been going on in his life that led to his decision to come to a group. He has worked hard all of his life, and claims to have pretty well attained everything that he always wanted, but he is not very happy. I ask him what he means by having "everything that he always wanted." Charles explains that he is married to his high-school sweetheart, has two children (a boy and a girl), owns his own business, attends church on a regular basis, and is well regarded in his home community. What does he mean by "not being happy?" He says that he is often depressed, that he has become lazy and lacks motivation. He "just can't seem to get the energy anymore." I agree with him that this would be very confusing. He had set out in life believing that all he had to do was what he had, in fact, done; but now that he has accomplished what he set out to do, it isn't enough—he still isn't happy.

We discuss what he has done to try to resolve this problem. He says that he has tried everything he can think of—going to church more often, taking extra days off, talking to his wife about it, cutting down on his bad habits, even trying out another relationship for a while. For information, I ask what he means by "bad habits." Charles admits that he smokes about a pack of cigarettes a day, swears a bit, and goes out drinking with the boys once or twice a month. I ask if he gets drunk those nights, to which he answers, "No." Then I ask, "How did all those things you tried work out for you?"

"Not very well, obviously!"

My next questions are, "Did they help you get what you want? For that matter, what do you want?"

Charles says that he wants to get on in life, to try to make some sense of what has gone wrong. At this point it is helpful to have a specific picture of what "getting on" might look like. When I ask, Charles shares that he has always wanted to learn to fly a plane. I ask him, "What would it mean to you to learn to fly a plane?"

"I would feel like I had accomplished something, and I would feel free."

"So, if you felt that you had accomplished something and felt free, what would that mean to you?" Charles states that he would then be happy. "Is that what you really want, to be happy?" Charles agrees.

We have now arrived at the final stage of Charles's introduction. I ask him if we can start to find a way for him to get what he wants, which is happiness, during this group process, how would that be? Charles answers emphatically, "Wonderful!"

For Janet, another member of our group, the scenario at the beginning of her introduction looks a lot different. Janet states her name, that she is twenty-one years old, has one child, is not married, and that she is a recovering drug addict and bulimic. The father of her child is also addicted and Janet describes herself as "co-dependent, on top of everything else!" She dropped out of college, has never held a real job, and is now living with her mother who is always telling her what to do. Janet's self-description includes statements to the effect that everything she has ever tried has failed and that everything seems hopeless.

I ask Janet what she has done, so far, to try to resolve her problems. She states that she has been attending a twelve-step recovery program for two years, but it has not been getting her anywhere. In addition, she has tried several types of counseling, none of which have ever worked. Everything she tries fails. She tried going back to school, but that didn't work out because she couldn't find a baby-sitter and her mother would not look after her son. She tried finding another place to live, but no one thought she should be out on her own, so she has given up on that idea. She tried to get her son's father to provide her with some support money, but she couldn't find him. Besides, whenever he was around, she usually got into more trouble. They would go out again for awhile until they started to fight. Then he would take off and she still wouldn't have any money for support. As I did with Charles, I ask Janet to evaluate how all these different attempts to improve her situation had worked out for her. From my viewpoint they obviously weren't effective at all, and even Janet had admitted already that they were not working, but the question is extremely important and needs to be asked in just those terms. "So, Janet, I can certainly see you have tried many ways to resolve all the things going on in your life. How have they been working out for you?" The answer is, as expected, "Not well at all!"

I then ask Janet what she wants. Janet's reply is that she simply wants to be happy. "What would *happy* look like to you?" Janet states that all she wants is to get a job, get a new boyfriend who understands her, move out of the house, and get her college diploma. "If you had all of that," I ask, "what would that mean to you?" She replies that then she would feel like she had more control in her life. "And if you had more control in your life, what would that mean to you?" Janet says that she thinks then she would be more at peace and feel strong.

"If we could find a way to start getting you what you want, and you could feel peaceful and strong, how would you like that?"

Janet's answer is, "Of course I'd like that a lot!"

Another example is Laurel. During her introduction to the group, Laurel states, among other things, that she wants to be a better mother. I ask her if she knows what a "better mother" would look like. Laurel isn't sure, but says she is interested in finding out. I ask her if she loves her daughter, to which she replies, "Of course." Next I ask whether she thinks that someone who loves her children is already a good parent. When she answers, "Yes," I ask her one more question. "Suppose you do not have to become a better mother? Suppose you are already a good mother? Suppose that all you really have to do is change a few behaviors? All you have to do is start doing some things that you have wanted to do? How would that be?" I could see a light come on. All of a sudden Laurel was not someone who didn't measure up—she was someone who only had to change a few of the things that she was doing to get what she really wanted.

These examples are slimmed-down versions of the introductions that I do for everyone in a group. Besides asking questions myself, I encourage other members of the group to ask questions too. Not all introductions have the immediate impact that Laurel's had on her, but the potential for this to happen exists during every introduction session.

It may seem that the way we arrive at what the clients want ignores a lot of important information about them. From the outset the entire approach of the Solution Group is that we are there to find solutions to the problems or challenges that the group members see in their lives. I never spend the introduction time digging into their pasts or wringing confessions out of anyone. My experience is that whatever information is needed will come forward, if not during introductions then at some other time as the group progresses. The information obtained during introductions can be supplemented, if necessary, by reference to available files, referral sources, or through individual counseling sessions.

There is no doubt that everyone in the group has been trying many things to control the outcomes of their various challenges. Charles experimented with several behaviors, from increasing church attendance to having an extra-marital affair. Janet had tried all sorts of things to resolve her situation. By being so creative and determined to try different solutions, Janet demonstrated how smart her behavioral system really is. There should be little difficulty in leading her to some need-fulfilling behaviors, because she is already used to trying things.

My aim for both of these clients, as it is for all group members, is to get them to evaluate how their various behaviors have been working out for them, and to have them arrive at a conclusion about what they are looking for. You will note that I do not stop at what it is that they are looking for on a tangible level. Janet and Charles want a lot of specific things to happen. The important information is not in what these things are, but rather in what it would mean to Charles and Janet if they got them. Therein lie their Real Wants! Never have I had a group that wanted anything less than happiness, peace, contentment, strength, etc. In most standard groups the participants identify with each other on the basis of their shared miseries. Charles and Janet could identify, perhaps, at some common level of pain recognizing that they are both lonely. In the Solution Group, however, individuals identify with each other on the basis of the positive attributes they all seek, their Real Wants—happiness, peace, contentment, strength. The identification and bonding process between group members begins during the introductions as they recognize that they share similar goals.

When the group members have identified their Real Wants, the leader conveys the message, "While you are here, we can get you started on that." The Solution Group does not promise the members that their problems will be solved right away, but that they will learn how to work on solving their problems themselves. Accomplishing the changes necessary to realize their Real Wants takes time. Although complete success is rarely possible during the course of the Solution Group especially when it is conducted in a concentrated format on consecutive days, all the group members will experience some immediate, initial successes, thus beginning the process of change. The Solution Group gives them the tools and teaches them the tactics they can use to continue towards their goals.

Currently most of the groups I conduct are closed, but the Solution Group process was developed initially in an on-going group with open admissions whereby new clients entered each week. New clients can enter a Solution Group at any time without becoming lost in the process. In the case of open admissions, a brief form of the introductions is conducted when a new client arrives to acquaint the newcomer with the group members, as well as to elicit the preliminary information that the group leader needs about the new member. In addition, the experienced members of the group are asked to give some feedback and to evaluate how they are getting their wants and needs met in the group. This not only benefits the newcomer, it also provides the experienced group members with an opportunity to review how they are doing and to evaluate their own progress. Because many of the central questions— What do you want? How has that been working out for you?—are asked during almost every session, newcomers are rapidly acclimated to the on-going process. Clients are encouraged to commit to the entire process. With a closed group this means attending every session; with an open, on-going group this means attending long enough to have cycled through all the different stages. While many clients benefit from repeating the series of stages, they are not encouraged to stay with the group indefinitely. My goal is to have them move on, to reach a point where they no longer need the group.

FEELINGS
Stage Two

KEY QUESTIONS
What feelings have you had in your life that you didn't like?
How many hours a day are you dealing with feelings you don't like?
Which of the feelings on our list have you not felt?
Are your feelings the biggest problem you have?
How would you like to be feeling?

ACTIVITIES
Identifying and listing feelings that participants don't like having.
Discussion of FEAR as the root of these feelings.
Listing feelings that participants want to have.

To start the discussion about feelings I ask the group members what feelings they believe they have been struggling with. "Please name a feeling that you have had, sometime in your life, that you did not like having. It doesn't have to be something that you are feeling right now, although that may be included." Sometimes it helps to ask for feelings that they consider to be "unmanageable." The "all your life" aspect of the question takes the focus away from any sense of the client being wrong at the present time, and it keeps the tone of the discussion from being confessional. Clients, being very aware and sensitive, often wonder about their feelings. The way this question is asked allows them to discuss their feelings in a non-critical fashion. Most clients readily begin describing the feelings that have been causing them the most disruption and discomfort.

One at a time, each person is asked to name one or two feelings they have had that they do not like. Every client needs to contribute something to the list. The outcome is most valuable when the list contains a rich assortment of feelings, and when none of the group members can escape by thinking that the exercise has nothing to do with them personally. Full and equal involvement, whenever possible, is the ideal.

In our typical group, Robert, the rebellious teenager, describes having felt "angry." I write down Robert's answer for all to see on a chalkboard or a flip-chart. Visibly recording each person's answer is essential. While I'm writing Robert's answer on the board, I ask if anybody else has been feeling anger. Several others usually agree that they, too, have had the same feeling. I don't ask them to describe their anger, nor do I encourage them to describe what specifically has been causing the anger, although they may volunteer that at the time. The only time we examine a feeling carefully is when the client has trouble identifying it. For instance, although Robert quickly identifies anger, he has difficulty describing another feeling. He says that he often feels distant and remote from others, never quite in contact. He states that even when he is in a room with other people he feels alone. As a result of discussing this with the group, he agrees to call this feeling "isolated." I add it to the list on the board.

As we continue around the group, Janet, the self-described failure, says she feels "guilty." Again, we don't ask Janet to elaborate about what brought on her guilt. We just want her to name the feelings she has had that she does not like. Anita, a victim of abuse, states that she has often felt "fear." I write FEAR on the board in capital letters. (I'll explain why shortly.) We continue around the circle.

I don't force an answer out of anybody who has trouble coming up with a feeling that they can share. I take my time and allow the clients to do the same. Telling them that we will come back to them in a minute or two usually works well, but sometimes a person still has nothing to add. In such cases a feeling can usually be extracted with a little ingenuity. For example, Albert, who seems very uncomfortable in the group, says he's too numb to think of any feelings—so I add "numb" to the list on the board. Another way to discover feelings that the client may not be able to verbalize is to ask them to talk about what brought them into counseling in the first place. Usually, the client describes a crisis they have faced. Albert, for instance, describes how he had concocted a plan to commit suicide, but then had been unable to carry it out. After Albert finishes describing his crisis, I ask him what he had been thinking about during that time. He says he was thinking how his life was useless and how weak he was that he couldn't even commit suicide successfully. Then I ask him how he was feeling when he was thinking that way. Usually, this type of questioning will garner some results and the client may even describe a feeling that is not yet on the board. Albert guesses that he was feeling "hopeless." I add it to the list.

I take care to deal only with feelings at this particular time. Marge, well groomed and poised, says at first that she is "confused." I agree that she probably is confused, then ask her if she is talking of confused thinking or feeling? When she states that it is her thinking that is confused, I ask her how she feels when she is confused in her thinking. To this she replies, "Anxious," so that is what I write down on the list. By making an effort always to be precise, I help the group to begin thinking in terms of the separate components of total behavior right from the start.

Once everyone has contributed, the list looks something like this: angry, isolated, FEAR, guilty, resentful, lonely, failure, useless, stupid, anxious, weak, at fault, hopeless, and so on. My groups always come up with at least thirty different feelings that they have had and did not like. Groups seem to have an endless supply of ways to describe how miserable they have been feeling.

After the group members have added as many feelings to the list as they can think of, I make some inquiries into how the clients' feelings have affected their lives. It is important for the clients to express how they view themselves and their feelings. I start by asking the group, one person at a time, "How many hours a day are you dealing with feelings included on the list?" The time span can be compared to an eight-hour shift. "If you were getting paid for feeling like this, how many hours a day would you get paid?" Invariably one or two people, if not almost everyone in the group, reply that they spend anywhere from 12 to 20 hours a day somehow involved with these feelings. (That many clients have trouble sleeping at night accounts for what appears to be such extraordinarily high figures as 20 hours a day of feeling pain. The reason they are awake is they are feeling angry, guilty, or something else listed on the board!) From hours in a day, the next step is to ask them how many days a week they spend with these feelings. Long-suffering, fearful Anita figures it adds up to about eight days a week!

Ted, a reluctant member of the group, insists that he has such feelings only 15 minutes a day. Usually the clients who mention such a short time span are new to the group, but not always. They often revise their answers upward a second time through the exercise. Even when a client like Ted insists that he experiences these feelings only 15 minutes a day, I do not suggest that he might be lying. Clients take offense at such a critical approach. A better tactic is to say, "If you are experiencing these feelings only 15 minutes a day, that's great. I certainly wouldn't want you to feel more pain. However, let me ask you another question. Is 15 minutes of pain a day more than you want to feel?" Every time the answer has been "Yes." With this approach some of the resistance usually goes out of the client. The idea that the individual matters within the group setting and can have different answers is paramount. Each must be allowed his or her own viewpoint.

As noted above, when Anita offered the word "fear" in the group, I capitalized it. Having established our list and noted how seriously these feelings have affected the clients' lives, we now move on to a discussion of FEAR itself. As a group we talk of the nature of fear, fight or flight responses, etc. One day in group, quite a while ago, I suddenly realized that no one in the room really knew what fear was. When a group gets to this stage of the process, I always ask them, "What is fear?" I always get the same reaction —silence. So I quote the dictionary's definition: "A painful emotion caused by impending danger or evil," and infer from this definition that fear is simply a response to a threat. In control theory terms, when our needs are not getting met, we experience fear. A question I then ask someone in the group is, "Do you want to have fear?" The answer is always, "No." But when I next ask someone, "Do you want to be able to act on a threat?" The answer is invariably, "Yes." We don't take too long to discuss this paradox. The main point is that fear accompanies our perception of a threat. The threat does not have to appear real to anyone else, but it is a very "smart" system that perceives threat and attempts to remove that threat. Fear itself is not a difficulty; it is only a problem when we are unable to deal effectively with whatever threat is the source of our fear, so that our feeling of fear continues.

Next I introduce the idea that fear is behind many of the other feelings the group does not like. As a group, we talk of the fear that is in the other feelings on the list. George feels lonely when he is *afraid* no one loves him or cares about him. Marge feels jealous when she is *afraid* she is going to lose someone's love. Charles feels resentful when he is *afraid* someone else will get credit for his work. Robert feels angry when he is *afraid* someone else has the upper hand ("the best defense is a good offense"). Janet feels guilty when she is *afraid* that people who get to know her will think she is a bad person and won't like her. With consistent question ing and discussion, we connect fear to every feeling on our list.

Now we are at one of the important turning points for the group. I ask each person, in turn, "What is there on this list that you have *NOT* felt?" (Let me stress here that the wording of this question is extremely important. It needs to be asked exactly this way.) In almost every case the group members say that they have felt *every* feeling on the list at one time or another. In my experience, whenever anyone states that he or she has not felt all of them, they usually identify no more than two or three of the feelings as ones they have never had. Again, I never dispute the clients' feedback, except when it is obvious that the client may need to evaluate a little more. In such cases I suggest a situation I think may have occurred that could have stimulated such a feeling and ask how they felt. Sometimes, then, they admit to a feeling they have denied, but sometimes they don't. I do not dispute their evaluation, but it is important that they be given the opportunity to evaluate.

The importance of the question, "Which of these feelings have you *not* had?" cannot be overlooked. Without any coercion or criticism, this question gives individuals in the group the opportunity to safely admit how miserable they have been. The evaluations that follow are much more meaningful when the group members have grasped the full scope and range of their feelings.

So far in this stage we have established what emotions the clients feel and the amount of time they spend feeling that way. The next step is to find out how they regard this difficulty they're having with their emotions, to find out how successful they believe their means of coping have been. I ask, "Is it true that your feelings are the biggest problems that you have? If you could just somehow feel better, would everything be all right?" Asking this question now helps me to make the connections later with the thinking and doing components of total behavior. Invariably the group members will evaluate their feelings as being the single biggest difficulty in their lives. If they could only feel better then they could get a job, a new and improved relationship, or whatever they need. They would willingly accept almost any condition if they could feel better. It's amazing how this desire becomes a common bond among all the group members. It's an ongoing wish shared by almost everybody.

Having used the group process to help the clients discover what a profound role *feelings* play in their lives, I begin asking how successfully they feel they deal with their feelings. After they make a list of their feelings and tell what they have done until now to deal with those feelings, I ask them, "How has it been working out for you?" The reply is, "Not so good." I follow this with, "If you could live a life the way you wanted and feel better, how would that appeal to you?" Occasionally I get stunned looks from clients who don't realize that there is a different way to live than what they have become accustomed to.

The discussions about feelings usually take quite a while. The evaluative questions are left floating within the minds of the group members. "How is it working out for you?" may seem like an obvious question, but it is an essential, simple, and useful evaluation for the client to make. Another might be, "How would you like to be feeling?" It is never too early to ask. Their curiosity is piqued, and has prompted them all to state that they would like to find a better way to live, although most of them have no idea how or what that might involve. I allow time here to reassure clients that they can have pretty much whatever they want. Janet, for example, has said that she has spent her entire life trying to cope with the guilt she feels, and that she's never gotten anywhere.

"You have tried to stop feeling guilty. Right?"

"Yes."

"I wonder, other than trying to stop feeling guilty, what do you want to feel?"

"I want to feel peaceful."

We continue in the rest of the discussion to clarify some of these feelings that the clients want to have. We talk about what Janet wants, rather than what she does not want. Most often, group members have no idea what something like "peaceful" would look like, so we spend some time discussing that.

At this point I start a new list on the board, comprising all the feelings that the group members *want* to have. Again, everyone adds something to the list, which eventually includes peaceful, happy, serene, confident, assured, assertive, successful, attractive, and so on. As with Janet's desire to feel peaceful, we spend some time going over what these feelings might look like. I suggest, at this point, that it is possible for the group members to begin the process of feeling these emotions if they are interested. The choice is theirs. The road to recovery involves achieving the feelings that they want.

One or two clients, like Janet or George, will always say that they are more concerned about getting rid of the old feelings first. I agree with them, but then I say, "I know that you are all smart people and that you have tried to get rid of the old feelings before, right? What are some of the things that you have done?" Whatever they answer, I ask, "And how has that worked out for you?" When this line is pursued, the clients start to revise their point of view. For most of them, of course, it has not worked out at all.

I mention to the group my own attempts in the past to achieve a successful recovery. I use the example of my own loneliness to convey the idea of going for the challenge of getting to feel what you want instead of trying to get rid of the old. At one time I also felt that the only thing really wrong with my life was how badly I was feeling. If I could somehow feel better, I thought, then everything would be okay. The biggest specter in this haunted existence was the dreadful loneliness I felt. Being a

44

fairly bright person I knew that I was lonely and that I should do something about it. I spent many hours over several years locked away in my basement apartment meditating, reading, questioning, and feeling worse all the time. I did the best that I knew how at the time. The solution only came for me when I started to focus on what I wanted to be and how I wanted to feel rather than on what I wanted to get rid of. The group always asks me what I did. Instead of answering directly, I ask them, "If what I did—and still do—looks like it could get you what you want, would that interest you?" Of course it would. "I learned to focus on what I wanted, and I was willing to change the other things I was doing to get what I wanted. I came out of my basement, for one thing."

In the end we spend some time, though not a lot, on possible solutions to reaching their new challenges. It is difficult to arrive at solutions to unwanted feelings without involving the other components of total behavior which we have not yet discussed in group. It has taken much work just to get the group to the point where they all agree on the similarities in their feelings and their need to find better ways to cope with these feelings.

THINKING
Stage Three

KEY QUESTIONS

What are you thinking when you have feelings you don't like?

Have you ever thought you were stupid, a failure, etc., after something you've done?

If this is what you are thinking, how would you expect to feel?

If you were happy, what would you be thinking?

What could you do to start thinking that way?

ACTIVITIES

Thinking/Feeling Exercise

Discussion of "secret thinking"

Making choices to change thinking about oneself

In the previous session we determined that most of the clients believe their feelings are the biggest problem facing them in their lives. In addition, they believe there is nothing they can do to feel better, although their efforts continue. The aim in this stage of the process is to have the participants realize that how they feel is closely connected to what they are thinking about themselves and their lives. In addition, we pursue some ideas about whether it is possible to change our thinking and, if we can, how that is done.

Robert, for instance, always gets angry as a way of trying to meet his needs and get what he wants. He shouts and yells—at times he has punched holes in the wall. He has tried numerous times to stop getting angry. My question for him is, "I know that you're feeling angry, and I know you're hitting walls. What are you thinking about when you are doing these things?" During the entire group process, all group members are asked this question, or a variation, right from the start. Surprised, they often say, "What does it matter what I am thinking?" Because our behavior is total, we cannot independently do something without it registering on the entire behavioral system. When we act in ways that we ourselves find unlikable, it affects what we think of ourselves and, in the end, how we feel about ourselves.

As stated before, the group members are aware that their feelings need some work. They have gone to great lengths to try to deal with their feelings. The beginning of this stage is spent on taking a closer look at the clients' feelings and developing a connection between their feelings and thoughts. While it is an oversimplification to focus only on the thinking and feeling components of total behavior, it is an excellent place to start. Clients don't yet know about all the possible connections between the components of total behavior, so we begin at a level they can easily grasp.

The exercise that I use at this stage with the group is based on one that I learned during my basic week of training in control theory and reality therapy. Its purpose is to show participants the relationship between what they are thinking and what they are feeling. I instruct everyone to close their eyes, and then I ask them to do each of the following, in turn, allowing 10-15 seconds for each step:

1. Think of the color red.
2. Think of the color blue.
3. Think of the color yellow.
4. Stop thinking yellow.
5. Feel sad.
6. Feel happy.
7. Open your eyes and raise your right hand.

When done, I ask them a series of questions. The first is, "Which of the instructions was the easiest to follow?" They all say, "Opening my eyes and raising my hand." It required little or no thought and had no real feeling component. Next I ask, "If you got the color red, how did you do it?" Another way to ask the same thing is, "What did you think of to get the

48

color red?" Charles and Marge say they saw a stop sign, Albert says he saw a sunset. The particular way anyone sees the color is not relevant. Some, like Ted, say that they couldn't think of anything at all. I ask him if he tried. This is an important question. If Ted says he did not try, I simply reassure him and move on. Remembering that this is a non-critical environment is more important than trying to get a particular client to comply. I ask similar questions about the remaining steps. Usually people think of the sky or the ocean to get the color blue, and they will see the sun or flowers to get the color yellow. Expect a wide variety of responses. At the step, "Stop thinking yellow," I ask how many people were able to do it. Of those who answer positively, I ask how they accomplished it. They usually report that they went back to thinking of a previous color or forward to thinking of a new color, thus demonstrating the principle of thought substitution. It is not possible just to stop thinking something; it is only possible to start thinking something else.

In the area of feelings, the clients' thoughts may be quite graphic. A common theme which surfaces when they are thinking of something sad is a funeral of someone they have known. Anyone who does not want to do the sad or unhappy part is neither criticized nor prodded into it. Members of the group usually personalize this part of the exercise, so expect a few moments of "let-down." That is why I do this part of the exercise first, before the happy part. Ending with the happy feeling follows the guideline to always end on an upbeat note. If the group is left on the down note, that is where they may stay. Sometimes, when we do the part on feeling happy I can see people smiling, so I know when they have gotten the happy feeling from their thinking.

I then ask the group if they noticed anything in particular about the exercise as a whole. Generally, they don't know what I'm looking for, so I have to provide the answer myself. Those people who had the clearest thought or mental picture of what the color or feeling would be like were the ones who stated that they arrived at the color or feeling. Those who thought of stop signs clearly saw red, and so on. Those who came up with the funeral scenes felt sad. Those who thought of having fun with their children felt happy. Those who chose not to, or stated they could not think of anything sad or happy, did not get those particular feelings. By pointing this out, the clients begin to understand that their feelings and their thoughts are closely connected.

Some discussion follows about the relationship of thoughts and feelings. I ask them the old chicken-or-egg question, "Which comes first?" In the exercise that we have just done, thinking led to what we were looking for, whether it was colors or feelings. This is a little harder for some to grasp than others. To those having trouble making this connection, I say, "All your life you have been bothered by the feelings that we talked of yesterday. And all of your life you have tried to work on those feelings.

How has working on your feelings been working out for you?" The answer is always something like, "Not too well." Then I ask, "If there were something else that you could work on and somehow or other you would feel better, how would that be?" The usual answer is, "That would be great!" Next I suggest, "Suppose that one way to begin this process was to start looking at the way you are thinking, and your feelings might become more of what you are looking for. How would that be?" Every time that I have adopted this tactic, the clients have taken a closer look at the idea and at least given it more thought. We often take a break at this point, and I encourage everyone to come back and challenge this idea, that what we are thinking has a direct connection to what we are feeling.

Out of this exercise comes a discussion about the source of our feelings. Up to this point most of the group members fervently believe that the root of all their difficulties has been how they have been *feeling*, not what they have been *thinking*. For many years they have been trying to do something about their feelings, hoping that maybe they would feel better. The Thinking/Feeling exercise and our group discussions help them discover the close connection between their thoughts and feelings and to realize that they can change how they think about themselves. The basic principal is that of substitution —it is not possible to stop ineffective thinking; one must replace it with effective, positive thinking.

When I ask, "If I told you that you could stop feeling lonely, but never talk about or think about getting rid of loneliness, how would that sound," Albert's answer to this question is typical. Although he had hardly participated at all up to this point, he now challenges me. "No one can stop being lonely without working on loneliness!" I agree with him that it certainly looks that way.

I share with Albert and the group that I spent several years trying to get rid of my own loneliness, and the best I could come up with on my own did not work. I used to go home (where I was alone) to try to figure out how to stop being lonely. However, once I was willing to change other components of my behavior, including my thinking, the loneliness began to fade away. I ask Albert, "What if it is true, and you can find a way of not being lonely without focusing on loneliness? Would you be interested?" He says, "Of course!"

Now we examine what the clients have been thinking about themselves, what I call their "secret thinking." Clients usually have a whole lot of thinking going on that they don't want anyone to know about. One of the most common examples is the thinking that they are quietly (or not so quietly) going crazy. In my own past, perhaps the most damaging behavior that was going on was in my brain, where no one could see it. I certainly did not look as if I was doing anything but wasting away. Inside my brain, however, thoughts were rolling around and around. I refer to this type of thinking as "spin dryer thinking."

One area of secret thinking that we discuss as a group is "hidden rules" that we all live by. Many of my clients have extensive mental lists of things that they should or shouldn't be doing, along with the things they can't do or could have done. And, of course, one mustn't forget the musts and have-to lists that are also running in our heads. Too often, clients make successful attempts at changing their behaviors, but then, from somewhere, comes the thought that they should or could have done better —and there goes the benefits of their change. They are left with the idea that what they did was just not good enough. Many of the people coming into group have created an entire thinking process built around that one belief about themselves—that whatever they try is either not good enough or they should have done better. Continually comparing oneself to other people is equally damaging.

Unflattering names that people call themselves represent another sort of secret thinking. Discussion of these names is one of those times when self-disclosure by the group leader is very valuable. I had a private name that I used to call myself—Puke. If I can admit to having once thought of myself as "Puke," then the clients are likely to feel it's okay for them to disclose their own secret names. The leader's secret name need not be worse than those of the group member. Disclosing any unflattering name is sufficient to connect the leader with the group. As each member reveals his or her private name, I list it on the board. Often this process makes some members of the group uncomfortable. For those who are reluctant I try to soften the discussion by asking them if there was ever a time when perhaps they thought they were stupid, maybe after having made a mistake. Their acknowledgment of this is all that it takes to get them included in the exercise.

The question I now pose to the group is, "If this is what you are thinking, how would you expect to be feeling?" The dawn of understanding breaks. They have evidence before them that their thinking could be connected to how they are feeling. We haven't completed the entire process yet, but they have made an excellent start. The idea is tossed around that perhaps there is something else they can do besides just trying to feel better. Anita suggests that perhaps they need to think positively and then everything will be okay. I ask her if she has tried that before. She says she has, so I ask her how it turned out. She states, "Not worth a damn." How would it work out to do the same thing again? She chuckles, "Not worth a damn!" Then I ask Anita if she is interested in changing her thinking in a way that is meaningful for her, and she says, "Of course." The point here is to emphasize that this is not just a course on the power of positive thinking. The purpose is to make the clients aware of the new choices open to them if they desire effective and meaningful changes in their lives. These changes can affect their thinking and their feelings, if that is what they want.

Before this stage is complete, we make a list of what they want to think about themselves. We know that they are now thinking of themselves as losers, etc., but what do they want to think? The list of "want to's" for the group looks like this: attractive, useful, loving, lovable, compassionate, and so on. This list is fun to work on. Sometimes a client has trouble thinking of something to add to the list. Albert, for instance, says he has no idea. I ask, "If you were happy, what would you be thinking?"

"I'd be thinking I was okay."

I ask him if he has a picture of what "okay" would look like.

"Not really," he shrugs. So I ask him if he would like to find out what that picture of "okay" would look like. His answer is, "Sure."

"If you are 'okay,' what would you be doing?"

"I'd be back with my family."

"And if you were back with your family, what would you be thinking about yourself?"

"That I was someplace I belonged." "That I belong" becomes Albert's contribution to the list.

Lastly, we discuss what the clients can do to start making the changes in their thinking that will give them what they want. It is important to ensure that all clients choose something that is suitable to their wants, that will help meet their needs, and that will take them to where they want to go, instead of away from where they have been. For instance, rather than have Albert start to look at choices that will help him feel less lonely, we work on choices that will help him think about what he wants to think about himself. His choices could be reading or going out and doing something fun. At this point, the suggested solution should be small enough that he can easily accomplish it. In the case of addicted clients who are attending Alcoholics Anonymous or another recovery program, it is sometimes quite easy to come up with activities to help take their thinking where they want it to go. Suggestions can include going to meetings, getting a sponsor, or reading the book *Alcoholics Anonymous*. With other clients, ideas may be more difficult to come by, but if you can get to know your clients, the job becomes easier.

The idea conveyed at the end of this session is that if you can at least start changing your thinking behavior, maybe you can start to feel better. I continue to caution people that this process is not about trying to better your thinking, and it is not about making yourself a better person. It is about starting to think about yourself in a positive way! While some may consider this merely a matter of semantics, stating the goal in these terms maintains the non-critical atmosphere of the group. After completing this stage, one overweight client described the shift in her thinking by saying, "I've decided I am done with dieting; now I'm into decorating what I've got!" Her glowing smile and regal posture emphasized how attractive she felt!

ACTIONS
Stage Four

KEY QUESTIONS
What have you been doing that you do not like doing?
Is it helping you get what you want?
Which of the actions on the list have you not done?
What do you want to be doing?

ACTIVITIES
Compiling a list of unwanted actions
Discussion of how actions are purposeful
Listing things the clients want to be doing

After dealing with the feeling and thinking components of total behavior, we move to the *doing* component, or actions. We follow the same routine, more or less, that we have followed so far. It seems to help the process along when the clients become accustomed to a regular flow in the sessions. As in previous meetings, the clients have a chance to review their behavior and evaluate their actions. The eventual outcome helps tie in their actions with the thinking and feeling components of their behavior.

I start the group off by asking, "What have you been doing that you do not like doing?" The behavior can be anything, no matter how long ago the event might have occurred. As in all the group sessions, we go slowly and include all the members of the group. All the unwanted actions are written on the chalkboard so everyone can see them. Occasionally someone mentions a thought or a feeling. If this happens, I stop and ask if what they have said represents *thinking, feeling,* or *doing.* An exchange with Robert demonstrates how this works. In answer to the initial question, Robert states that one thing he has been doing is getting angry.

"That's okay," I say, "but is getting angry an action or a feeling?"

"A feeling, I guess."

"What do you do when you get angry?"

"I shout and yell a lot."

Shouting and yelling are the actions I add to the list. As before, the group members are gently guided to recognize and distinguish the different components of their total behavior.

All group members make at least one contribution to the list of behaviors. I go as slowly as necessary, using many of the tactics I employed when we compiled the previous lists of feelings and thoughts that they didn't like having. The list of unwanted actions includes shouting, arguing, lying, swearing, slamming doors, hitting people (and other violence), crying, getting revenge, stealing, withholding or demanding sex, blaming, gossiping, smoking, bullying, cheating, drinking, doing drugs, and the list goes on. One behavior that I always like to get on the list is "P.I. work," which stands for "Private Investigation" work, the term I use to describe how people check up on others when they don't believe them. Marge, for instance, reveals that she came to the group seeking help after one of her "P.I." trips went awry and she used a golf club to smash in a windshield. It is not unusual to have every group member own up to P.I. activity in the midst of nervous laughter. Marge is much relieved to find other trackers in the crowd. Groups seem to get a chuckle from this whole discussion.

Having completed the list to the satisfaction of the group, we then discuss what these actions are all about. The conviction that their actions get them into an awful lot of trouble is universal among my clients. Even Ted, who doesn't seem too involved yet, agrees that he is not getting the results he is looking for by going to jail. For many of my clients, repeated episodes of drinking, thieving, violence, and so on, are "usual," but they are not the acknowledged goals of a lifetime. We go back over some of the admitted actions of individual group members.

What they are often looking for is the thread that will make sense out of what they have been doing. "Why?" holds a prominent place in the minds of group members.

I usually start off by asking the members if they are aware of the reason behind their actions. It is imperative at this time to point out that what they did in the past, or are still doing now, does not have to make any sense to them or the rest of the world. That is not to say that there is no reason for what they do. This is usually a totally new proposition to them. By way of explanation, I start off by challenging everyone to think of one day in their lives that, given the information they had at the time, they did not do their best. The crucial part of this is "given the information they had at the time." Someone will always say, "But I should have known..., or thought..., or done...." I remind them that they didn't know that, or think that, or do that—so what they did was probably the best they could have done at that particular time. A good example to use here is an alcoholic client who intended to stay sober, but repeatedly went back to the bars he got drunk in (even when he was "on the wagon") because that was where his friends were. Inevitably, despite his desire to stay clean, he would slip back into drinking, because at times of crisis, drinking was his means of coping. The question is, did he really *know* how dangerous the time he spent in the bars was? In fact, at the time, he did not.

This is the point in the process where control theory/reality therapy concepts about basic needs are interjected. At every step along the way it is paramount to educate. The key idea here is simply that when our needs are not getting met, we behave in a way that will meet those needs, even if we do not like some of the things we do. The list of actions the group has compiled, like their lists of feelings and thoughts, exemplifies the variety of activities that we try to get our needs met. Nothing, short of death, will ever stop us from trying.

I then introduce the group to the five basic needs, identified by Dr. William Glasser, that we are all constantly striving to satisfy—*Love/Belonging, Achievement/Power, Freedom, Fun,* and *Survival*. We talk about what each one means. I introduce the acronym L.A.F.F.S. to help the group to remember them. Many people are more comfortable talking about "belonging" instead of or in addition to "love" if the word "love" has predominantly romantic or sexual connotations to them. Similarly, although Dr. Glasser uses the term "power," the word "achievement" seems to work better in the Solution Group, because the word "power" for many people has negative or political implications. It is important to point out that the ability to make choices is fundamental to the concept of "freedom." Everybody knows what fun is, at least for themselves! Survival —our physical needs for food, water, shelter, etc.—is the need that group members accept most easily as essential, but it is usually not difficult to get even skeptics to accept, at least as a working hypothesis, that psychological needs are essential also. As we continue to talk in group about the basic needs and how to meet them, their understanding will deepen.

At this point in the group process I do not try to develop specific correspondence between the clients' actions and the particular needs they are trying to meet, but I do introduce them to the concept that all our behavior represents our best attempt, at the time, to meet our basic needs. We talk about the effects that their undesirable actions have on the other areas of their lives. Typically a client such as Robert may state that he is unhappy with his shouting behavior. He may say he *feels* "guilty" about his actions and *thinks* that he's not able to control himself very well. The next questions for him are, "How are those thoughts and feelings working out for you? And are they helping you get what you want?" Robert should then identify what exactly it is that he wants. The client and the group are all a part of this evaluation, which is one of the most important features of the Solution Group process. During every step of the way each person evaluates his or her own behavior and gets to hear the self-evaluations of their fellow group members. (I interrupt any interpersonal attacks by group members by asking, "How is saying that helping you get what *you* want?" This maintains the non-critical, non-judgmental atmosphere of the Solution Group and emphasizes the importance of *self*-evaluation, not evaluation of others.)

We also talk during this stage about the controlling nature of these behaviors, how they are purposeful in the sense of being attempts to meet our needs or get us what we want. Since violent behaviors are always on the list, we talk of how violence can be purposeful. As long as a behavior is effective, in that it seems to get a person what he or she wants, the behavior will be used again and again. Many behaviors stop when they no longer have any value to the person doing them. In the case of the abusive parent, violence may seem beneficial until one day the child turns on the abuser and the price of abusing becomes too high to continue. There are many examples in our society of times when those around us have reformed. Some addicts, for instance, eventually decide that they have had enough of an old behavior, that they are no longer getting their needs met through their addictions. (Fortunately for them, meaningful direction and assistance is available through Alcoholics Anonymous and similar programs.) It is a good practice in group to go through all the actions on the list, showing how each of them is purposeful and how they may not get us what we really want, but they do provide us with something. Usually this discussion brings out still more undesirable activities!

After this full discussion, I usually pick the toughest nut in the room and ask, "What is on the list that you have *NOT* done?" (As with the list of feelings they didn't like, it is crucial to ask this

63

question exactly this way.) This is the point when one would expect to see widespread evidence of denial among all of the members. If most of these people were asked directly to tell about their lying, or their abusing, or their stealing, they would quite likely deny to some degree that they engaged in such behaviors, or admit to some only reluctantly. This particular question is amazing because even though the group has compiled an extensive and varied list of disagreeable actions, the clients rarely identify more than one or two actions as ones they have NEVER done! Ted, who had told the group his father was abusive and violent, accepts the list and thereby admits that he himself has been abusive and violent. Laurel, the battered wife of an alcoholic, admits that she herself has used drinking to try to feel better and has "slapped her kids" in anger. Charles, who represents himself as a pillar of the community, agrees to everything on the list, including threatening suicide. In short, this process levels the playing field with any mix of clients. No coercion is used. No person is forced to admit doing anything he or she hasn't done or doesn't want to admit doing. But admit it they do!

It is important to note that we don't dwell on these past actions. The process of evaluation continues. The group members, collectively and individually, are asked to evaluate how their life-styles have been working out for them. We stay with the evaluations until everyone understands and has made some assessment of how things have been going for them. It is important to make the evaluative process meaningful for the client, so the alcoholic client needs to evaluate his or her drinking behavior, the abused client needs to evaluate her co-dependency, the parolee his criminal behaviors, etc. If you have any question as to the possible dishonesty of the responses, you can continue to probe with further evaluative questions, but in the end the responsibility for honesty remains with the client, and their evaluation needs to be accepted.

One of the analogies that I use in the group that helps to explain the uselessness of trying to "fix" behaviors is comparing ourselves to an outdoor Christmas tree that is still alive but weak and spindly, in need of nourishment. The behaviors that we exhibit are the decorations on the tree—our attempts to look better. We all end up with several dozen unattractive decorations, including guilt, hate, anger, shouting, procrastination, depression, and thinking that we are losers, unattractive, and so on. Routinely we try to fix these behaviors. From day to day we continuously and routinely take a decoration or even several and try to "shine them up," hoping somehow that when we are done we will have new, pretty decorations and be a good-looking tree. Unfortunately, if these are the only decorations that we have, shining them up is not enough to make us good-looking trees. What we want is to be a healthy tree decorated with effective behaviors!

We have simple requirements. All that we need to flourish is to have our needs met. The water that we use contains love, achievement, freedom, fun and survival, and if we are careful about watering ourselves, we will continue to grow stronger and healthier. If we do not allow ourselves to meet these simple needs, then our tree becomes overwhelmed and weakened by all the worrisome, tarnished decorations of ineffective behaviors. In my own life, I have not totally eliminated any of my ineffective behaviors, but I have learned to meet my needs and have decorated myself with new, effective behaviors. When I use this analogy in a group, most people grasp it very easily. In only a few minutes some of the group members begin referring to their behaviors as "just another decoration." They begin to see through this simple tool. Learning to meet their needs and choosing effective behaviors is the challenge, not fixing or "shining up" ineffective behaviors.

Now is usually a good time to discuss guilt. Time after time, individuals want to hang onto their guilt—it's a "decoration" they think they ought to have. At the same time that they are insisting they should keep it, they are also trying to get rid of it! It's surprising how many people, such as Marge, believe that guilt is a useful and fulfilling feeling, at least to some degree. Before coming to the group, Marge had been very successful in her work, but had not yet had a successful relationship. She had married two alcoholics and had a son who was also alcoholic. She could not keep her mother happy. She felt very guilty—if only she had been a better wife, mother, and daughter, then all these other people would have been happier. The desire to become a "better" person was the motivation behind her joining the group. I ask her, "How is all that guilt working out for you?" She replies that she doesn't like the feeling but believes it is helping her. "What benefits do you get from the guilt?" Marge's answer is about the best that anyone can come up with, "It helps me stop doing the bad things I was doing." We then talk about the difficulty of "stopping bad things" without substituting "good things" that help to meet one's needs. "Do you really need guilt to prod you into doing good things?" Guilt can be dealt a crushing blow by having the group evaluate exactly who benefits from guilt. They soon begin to see that guilt serves only other people and not themselves. This guilt business pops up frequently, and it always bears attending to since most clients cling to it. The offer of a new point of view, making their own choices, appeals to them.

Once all the clients have made their assessments about their undesirable actions, understand the basic needs, and are primed to start looking for new ways to meet their needs, the next question is, "So, if this is what you have been trying and it has not been getting you what you want, what do you want to be doing?" The group now compiles another list that looks like this: honest, self-reliant, peaceful, trusting, open-minded, accepting, spiritual, loving, attractive, confident, compassionate, and assertive. You may notice something peculiar about this list. When asked to describe behaviors that they did not like doing, the group members were very specific. They mentioned shouting, lying, cheating, stealing. When asked what they *want* to be doing, however, they are much more vague. Also interesting is how much this list resembles the lists of how they want to feel and what they want to think of themselves.

When the new list has been made, I ask the group to tell me what these behaviors would look like. Most often I get a blank stare. It seems as if they have all these ideas of how they want to be acting, yet have no idea about how it might look. Because all of our behavior is purposeful, and when we are behaving we are all headed in the direction of what we want, it helps to have a good idea of what it will look like when we get what we want. I cannot fathom trying to get somewhere if I don't know the direction, or if I don't know what it will look like when I get there. I talk about "honesty" as an example. Usually the clients see the activity of "telling the truth" as a measurable part of "honesty." Then I have each client pick one item from the list of behaviors they want to be doing and come back to the group and tell everyone what it would look like. In other words, if they were being "successful," what would that look like? What would "confident" be like? "Trusting?" In their quality world pictures of their lives, what would they be doing, thinking, and feeling? An entire session can be spent on the descriptions they bring back.

When doing this activity, the leader should listen for comments that are of the "don't want" variety. Quite often, the clients build their pictures on what they *don't* want. Reality therapy training teaches the skill of asking the following simple question: "We know what you don't want. What is it that you do want?" Sometimes the clients say that they simply don't know what they want, at which time I ask them if they would like to find out. The answer is always, "Yes!" Then I usually ask them, "Do you know anyone who has what you want? What are they like?" Another thing to be alert for are the clients who say they want *more* of something. George, for instance, says if he were successful he would have more money. I pull a $5 bill out of my wallet, hand it to George, and say, "Great! Here is some *more* money. Are you successful now?" The point is that "more" has to be clarified; how much more is enough?

By now the group has discovered that although they have many so-called negative behaviors in common, they also have many positive wants in common. They want the same things, so now they work on the solutions together. They all agree that they would gladly be trying something different if they knew what they could be doing. A recovering addict may be familiar with what he needs to do for an ongoing recovery, but now he has a reason for reviewing his options. This exercise opens the minds of everyone in the group to the possibility of making choices that will get them what they want.

PHYSIOLOGY AND TOTAL BEHAVIOR
Stage Five

KEY QUESTIONS
In what ways have activities that you haven't liked doing affected your physiology?
How would your life look if things were the way you wanted?
What is something you can do to help you get what you want?

ACTIVITIES
Connecting actions with physical symptoms
Analyzing the "Control Car" model of total behavior

The remaining component of total behavior that the group has yet to discuss is physiology. For many clients, headaches, stomach disorders, or other health problems are the primary reason they sought help in the group, but every client can relate behaviors to physical outcomes. I remind the group of the several lists we have compiled: Feelings (depression, fear, anger, loneliness, resentment, etc.), Thoughts (self-blame, self-pity, name-calling, etc.), and Actions (drinking, swearing, hitting, lying, and many others). My first question for the group in this stage is, "What are some of the activities you have done which you do not like and which affected your physiology?" I use the word "physiology" instead of "health" on purpose, because I want them to concentrate on physical health, not mental health, and it helps maintain a non-judgmental atmosphere if we can discuss physical outcomes without implying they are good or bad, healthy or unhealthy. As in previous sessions, each member of the group is asked to contribute to the discussion by mentioning at least one activity along with an accompanying physical outcome. The only restriction I impose is that the activity and outcome must pertain to themselves. If a person mentions smoking, for instance, it must be their own smoking that they are talking about. This guideline forces each person to make a connection between their own behavior and physiology and helps maintain the non-critical, non-judgmental atmosphere of the group.

Clients have little difficulty understanding the question and supplying a wealth of examples. Charles says his continuous hacking cough is probably due to his smoking. George, an alcoholic, states immediately that his drinking gives him hangovers. In addition he attributes his being overweight to excess beer consumption and says that his stomach ulcer, too, is probably related to his lifestyle. Janet ties her bulimic behavior of overeating and disgorging food to her bad teeth, malnutrition, and listlessness. Marge complains of sleeplessness and an itchy rash, but isn't sure what activities of hers might be related, other than having a general feeling that they may be due to stress. When I ask her to describe her life at work she admits that she often worries a lot about meeting deadlines, drinks "gallons" of coffee, and resents her co-workers most of whom she characterizes as incompetent or lazy. She quickly recognizes the connection between worrying, caffeine consumption, and sleeplessness, but she doesn't connect the itchy rash until she remembers how it cleared up during her last vacation, only to reappear shortly after her return to work. These evaluations are representative but far from exhaustive. Most individuals find it relatively easy to connect actions to physiology. Connecting thoughts and feelings to physiology is sometimes more difficult, but most groups are able to identify tiredness or exhaustion as physical outcomes of worrying, guilt, and anger.

By this point in the process the group members are ready to start making connections between the various components of their behavior that they have identified. Although the clients have been involved all along in an education about control theory and reality therapy concepts, it has not been obvious. To tie the information together, I now present an educational activity that provides them with a way of making sense of it all. We talk about the relationships among all the various components of behavior that we have so far focused on individually by comparing our total behavioral system to a car, using Dr. Glasser's model (mentioned in the first chapter) to demonstrate the central concepts that all behaviors are connected and that one's feelings and physiology are often directed and powered by one's thoughts and actions. The "Control Car" looks like this.

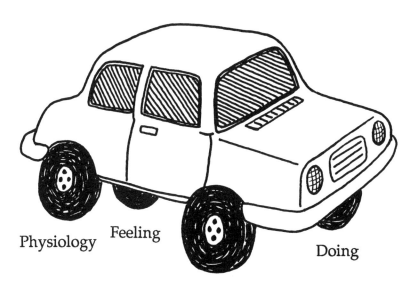

Physiology   Feeling

Doing

Thinking

There are a few key points to make when discussing the car as a model of total behavior. Our total behavior comprises four components: feeling, thinking, doing, and physiology. Each component affects the others, but two of the components, thinking and doing, dominate or "power" the others, much like a car with front-wheel drive (with the power and the steering located in the front wheels). In the car model of control theory, the two front wheels represent the thinking and doing components, because what we do and think will affect, if not dictate, our feelings and our physiology. An ideal example is the use of drugs or alcohol. Using these chemicals to feel good affects what we do, think, feel, and our health. It is hard to decide which of these areas is affected the most, because they are all tied in so closely. We then discuss all the behaviors that brought the various participants into the group. Anita, a chronic worrier, can identify the effects that worry has on her total behavior. She talks of resultant headaches, procrastination, and feeling strung out. Janet connects her eating disorder to feeling out of control, being secretive, and thinking that she is too fat.

Many of my clients are what I call "Thinkers," people who spend huge amounts of time trying to analyze their way out of their respective dilemmas. They believe that if they could just figure out what to do, everything would be great. Quite often, the Solution Group is not their first try at recovery. George told us he had tried over thirty sources—

counselors and workshops and such—in seven years. Marge said she had done a lot of reading to try to solve her problems. When I asked her how many self-help books she had acquired, she said, "Seven cartons!" Anita told me she had had several years of therapy, but no one ever suggested that perhaps all her analyzing was having disastrous effects on the rest of her life. In effect, the result of her constant thinking, analyzing, and worrying behaviors was an inability to function at any other level. When the group discussed the car model of total behavior, she realized that her thinking "wheel" was so large that it was having disastrous effects on the other components of her behavior. Anita's "Control Car" looked like this:

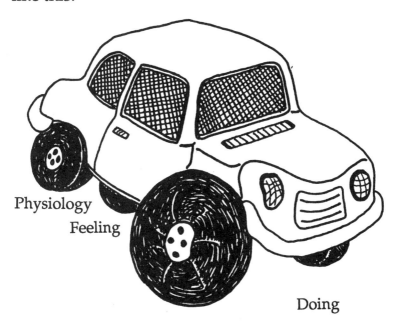

Physiology

Feeling

Doing

Thinking

The process of self-evaluation continues. Each person in the group evaluates the relationships among his or her behavioral components according to their own circumstances.

Another area that we touch on in this exercise is the cyclic nature of behavior. Old behaviors are repeated with the same result again and again. When our needs are not getting met, we will use whatever behaviors we can to meet them. If we have a limited repertoire to choose from that includes only negative behaviors, then we will select negative behaviors every time we try to meet our needs. By repeating the cycle we never get to what we really want. Once we have a new list of more effective behaviors to choose from, and those behaviors look meaningful to us, we will begin to substitute them for the ineffective, negative behaviors. Only when the clients start to adopt effective behaviors will they break the old cycles and get their lives headed in a new direction that will, eventually, get them what they really want.

As mentioned previously, the clients are looking for new things to do in their lives. They are in the Solution Group because what they have been doing has not been getting them what they want. Even those who adamantly deny serious problems are willing to admit that their lives are not perfect—something brings them to group. They are already aware that they will have to do something different to get what they want. They are, in fact, already doing something different simply by being in the room with the rest of the group.

Knowing that, I assume that they can at least take a new look at future options. I am always careful to allow them the freedom to choose between trying to do something new or going back to their old behaviors. However, I ask them to evaluate the natural consequences of their old behaviors if they plan on continuing them. The clients readily relate to the idea that by repeating their actions, whether it be stealing, abusing others, or drinking, they are guaranteeing that their "car" will continue in the same direction, never getting them to where they really want to go. They also realize that if they are always doing what other people want them to do, they are "giving away the keys to their car" and have no control over the direction of their own lives.

We wind down this topic by imagining how the ideal or quality car would look and what it would drive like. Each group member has some idea of how his or her life would look if things were the way he or she wanted. Sometimes individuals may claim that they don't have any ideas, in which case I slow down again to draw the person out, thus being sure they are included in the process.

Before going on to the next stage, we discuss specific behaviors that the group members can do to start getting them what they want. Generally, these are repeated from the previous sessions, but not always. Every group session brings new insights. Every day in the Solution Group the clients learn a lot, but if we don't move away from the problems to solutions they choose, then they have only been further educated about their pain. The process is intended to leave them with the idea that there are alternatives to their old behaviors.

BEHAVIOR AND RELATIONSHIPS
Stage Six

KEY QUESTIONS
How has your behavior affected your relationships?
What are your best interests, and where are you in relation to them?

ACTIVITIES
Diagramming relationships as affected by client's behavior
Self-evaluation of relationship between client's current behavior and the client's best interests

The next group activity helps the clients start to evaluate their own relationships. Most of the time they are very confused about their friendships as well as their relationships with parents and spouse (or significant other). To begin, I show them a diagrammatic way to represent their relationships.

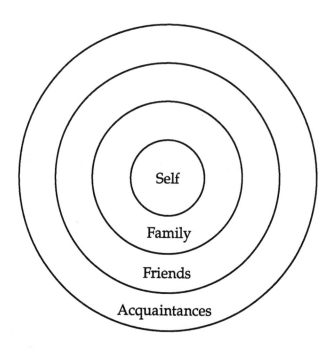

The above concentric circles, I tell them, represent the usual arrangement for relationships. I am careful to use the word "usual" in the group discussion. For most clients it seems to be more neutral and comfortable than the word "normal." Clients agree quite readily about what represents usual, but they express many divergent opinions about what constitutes normal. Furthermore, when clients get to the point of analyzing their own relationships, characterizing oneself as *unusual* is preferable to admitting that one is abnormal.

The group members accept the premise that usually family members are closest to us, then friends, and so on. Part of the same activity is to evaluate how our various behaviors (the ones identified as those we do not like doing) have affected and continue to affect our relationships with others. We include total behavior now—Doing, Thinking, Feeling, and Physiology. As a model, I draw the scheme for an alcoholic:

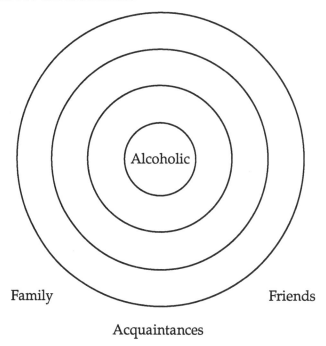

Family   Friends

Acquaintances

Alcoholics often feel removed from close relationships and speak of not feeling connected or not fitting in. This activity for analyzing relationships gives them the opportunity to start making sense of the influence that drinking and their thoughts have had on their lives. The evaluation is that the action of drinking is affecting their thinking and their feelings. As a result, the person who is addicted to alcohol feels and thinks that he or she is not close to anyone. If they feel that no one cares, their need for love or belonging is threatened. This calls for more need-fulfilling behavior, which in the case of the alcoholic will probably be more drinking, and the pattern of isolation is intensified.

The diagram for the alcoholic is similar to those of clients who persistently engage in various undesirable activities, but individual relationship maps drawn up by the clients incorporate many unique features. When clients first describe their relationships, however, quite often they stick to outward appearances or how they think they ought to look. I repeatedly remind them of the intent of the exercise and ask if the descriptions they are giving are as they think they should be or as they really are. During this process, all my counseling skills are used in coaching the clients to new insights.

This is not an exercise to evaluate how the behavior of others has affected the clients, which is a true turn-around for many of my clients who come into the group claiming that someone else is to blame for their difficulties. Often, as with Laurel, the co-dependent client's belief that someone else is to blame is so total that it is the driving force in their decision to get help. I never criticize a client for blaming others. They will catch on as they and others in the group do the self-evaluations. In open groups, the newcomers hear the more advanced members evaluate in a different way, which helps to shift their point of view.

Still another aspect of this activity is for the clients to evaluate what they have done to themselves through their own behaviors. I ask them how their behavior has affected their relationships with themselves. This usually gets blank stares. I rephrase the question. "If we are to perceive ourselves at the very center of our personal universe, would we be looking after our own best interests or not?" Having established the idea that we are indeed at the center of our own universe, we spend time on what that universe would look like if we were serving our own best interests.

Many clients have some difficulty distinguishing between selfishness and best interest. The guideline that I suggest is that our best interests are those things that we would want to be doing, thinking, or feeling, and that will help us get what we really want. The best interests that the group members come up with are such things as loving, caring, proud, humble, honest, attractive, and so on. I only collect three or four "best interest" words at this time and write them on the board. We will come back to this idea at the end of the session. If something is not going to help us get what we really want, then it is not likely to be in our best interest. If a client has some difficulty sorting this out, I help them evaluate whether or not a behavior is getting them what they really want. We discuss the idea of having our own best interests describe the "I" or "Me" in the middle of our lives.

At this point, we begin mapping out the existing relationships for each person in the group. We do so on the board for everyone to see. Usually the discussion so far has only started to open up the thinking of the group. Listening and seeing the maps develop expands the understanding for everyone in the group. To begin with, the concentric circles are empty. The client identifies people in his or her life and locates them at representative, relative distances from the center. Numbers are included when possible to indicate how many relationships of each sort the client has. Laurel's diagram, at this point of the proceedings, looks like the one below:

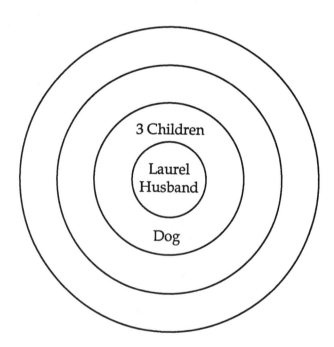

This diagram is typical of a co-dependent client who has entered the group as a result of someone else's behavior, or so they think.

When the client's relationship map is dramatically different from the "usual" one, the client is helped to evaluate how their behavior has affected their relationships. It is important, however, to be alert to unusual maps that reflect genuine cultural differences rather than patterns of ineffective behaviors. The relationship map drawn by a Japanese client, for example, shows family at the center and the self at the periphery, as below.

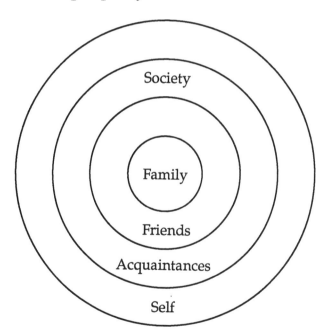

For someone raised in the Japanese culture, this represents the "usual" pattern of relationships;

the well-being of family is uppermost, even at the expense of one's own best interests.

Albert's map shows a combination of cultural influence and ineffective behaviors.

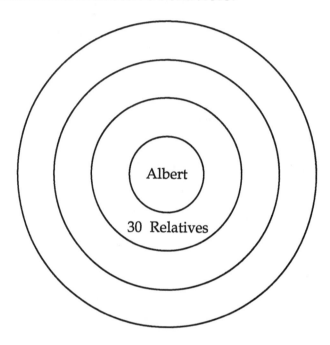

Albert's map indicates an unusually high number of family members, which is typical of his particular culture. Native Americans frequently consider extremely close friends among their family members, even to the point of calling people who are not true kinfolk "Auntie" or "Uncle." The importance of these individuals is the same as if they were relations by blood or marriage. On the other hand, Albert's map shows no relationships other than family, thus indicating the alienation and isolation he feels as a Native American living in an urban environment.

Charles, who has admitted to no particularly overwhelming difficulties in his life other than general unhappiness and dissatisfaction, initially draws a fairly usual relationship map.

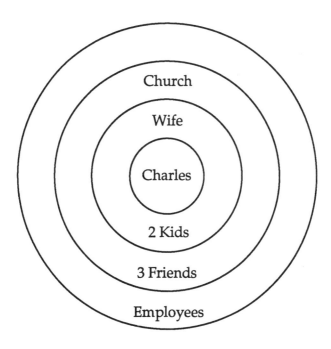

Remembering, however, that Charles admitted during the introductions to having had an affair, I ask him to re-examine how cheating on his wife affected his relationships. The new map that he draws shows a distinctly different pattern of relationships.

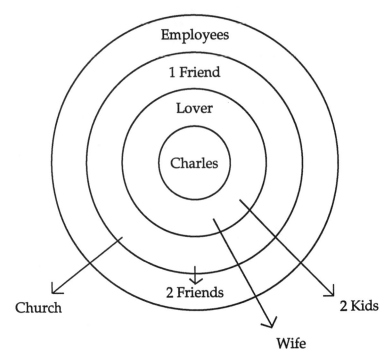

Employees

1 Friend

Lover

Charles

Church

2 Friends

Wife

2 Kids

Although during the time he was involved he felt quite close to the woman who was his lover, his deceit and guilt made him feel extremely distant from his wife, children, and church. Interestingly, Charles perceived no change in his relationship with the one friend who knew all about his extra-marital relationship, but he felt less close to other friends with whom he was not as honest. Analyzing how having an affair affected his relationships helps Charles to see why the affair had not been satisfying. It was an ineffective way to get what he really wanted.

After analyzing a client's relationships with other people, we turn to evaluating the client's relationship with himself, using the same diagrams. Ideally, our best interests will coincide with our "self" at the center of our universe, and at the center of the diagram. When I ask Laurel, "Where are your best interests on your map?", she says, as many others do, "Not even on the board!" So then I ask, "Where would your best interests be if not on the board?" Typically the response is, "On the floor," or something like that. I then give her a piece of paper, tell her to write her name on it, and ask her to put the paper where she thinks it goes in relation to the center of her own universe, represented by the center of the relationship diagram on the board. The clients now have some idea of how far out of tune they have been in relation to their own best interests. They have also begun to make the connection that their own behaviors are the source of their remoteness. When this exercise is finished, pieces of paper are scattered all around the room. Not all clients, however, put their name off the board, and it is not imperative that they do so. This is the client's own evaluation. But, when the idea is open that they can put their name anywhere, almost all opt for someplace far off the board. When discussing Albert's relationship map, I ask him to place his piece of paper somewhere that indicates how far from his family and his best interests his attempted suicide had put him. Without saying a word, Albert walks out of the room, goes down the hall, and leaves his name outdoors!

The next step is to modify the individual relationship maps to show how the clients would like
them to be. These new maps are called "quality
maps," because in control theory terms, they are
intended to represent the clients' quality world or
mental pictures of how their lives would be if they
had what they really want. Laurel's quality map
looks like this:

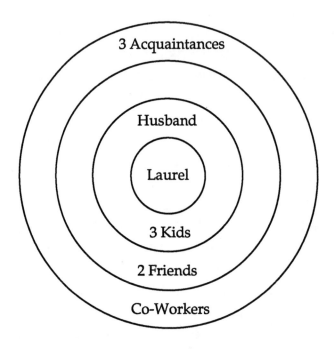

Moving her husband out of the center is
crucial for Laurel. Having another person so close as
to be indistinguishable from oneself is not an
effective relationship in the long run. Laurel's quality
map also shows relationships outside the immediate
family circle, which are important additions.

At this point, having established what their quality maps would or could look like, we expand our list of "best interests." I ask, "If you are back in the center of your world, what are some of the things that are in your best interest?" Usually the lists vary only slightly from group to group, but the group leader should be sure it includes certain key elements. With alcoholics, for instance, one would not want to give up on the list until the word "sober" was on it; with addicts the word "clean" should be there. The same idea applies for any special interest that pertains to the group. We discuss an interesting phenomenon. You may have noticed that the list of "best interests" and the "wants" that were listed earlier are very similar. In fact, they are essentially identical! Not only do the clients want to be attractive, smart, healthy, happy, and so on, it turns out that those are the very things that they believe are in their own best interests. "It's a pretty smart system," I point out, "that wants to be happy, healthy, and so on, when it is in its own best interest to be these very things! That means every person in this room is pretty smart." They have, by completing this process with their own wants and best interests, branded themselves as "smart people."

The final activity in this stage is to discuss the actions and behaviors that will help the clients establish their quality worlds. Usually they have done this before, because every session comes down to the process of arriving at possible solutions. The last minute or two before we break is spent on a blatant ploy to suggest how simple the process of recovery can be. I simply say, referring to the scraps of paper lying around on the floor, "Those of you who are interested in picking up your lives may now do so by picking up your names." Admittedly the recovery process is not that easy, but a simple decision to put oneself back into the center of one's universe can lead to dramatic changes. Laurel, for instance, went home after doing this exercise and refused to allow further abuse. Her husband threatened to come down and beat me up. I said, "Send him down!" He came—and ended up joining the group, saying he wanted to know what his wife had done so that he could do it too!

NEEDS AND RELATIONSHIPS
Stage Seven

KEY QUESTIONS
What do you think you have been doing to get your needs met?
What needs are being met by your relationships?
What could you do instead to meet your needs?

ACTIVITIES
Using the Needs Circle to chart behaviors and relationships which satisfy basic needs
Discussing ways to start to satisfy unmet needs

In the next session we continue to analyze the clients' relationships, but this time from the perspective of how they are meeting their needs. We review the five basic needs—L.A.F.F.S.—and discuss how various relationships help to meet these needs, concentrating particularly on the needs of Love, Achievement, and Freedom. I de-emphasize the need for Fun at this stage, because clients are too quick to latch on to a lack of "Fun" as the root of all their problems. In my experience, persons who satisfy their needs for Love, Achievement, and Freedom, rarely lack for Fun, and if they do, it is a relatively easy matter to resolve. Meeting the needs of Love, Achievement, and Freedom presents a greater challenge. The diagram I use to analyze how we meet our needs is called a "needs circle." The following diagram is the *usual* needs circle:

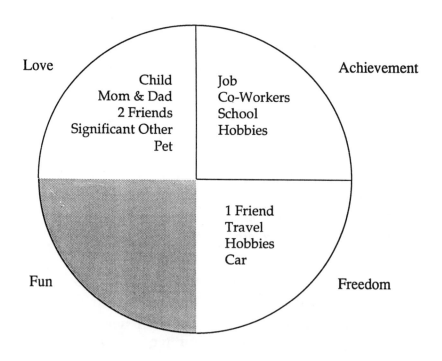

The needs circle resembles a pie cut into quarters, one each for Love, Achievement, Freedom, and Fun. The point of the activity is to evaluate the clients' relationships according to which needs they meet. Inevitably, we end up including activities and other things besides relationships on the clients' charts, but I prod the clients repeatedly to think about how their relationships meet their needs because they are unlikely to include them otherwise. The relationships should be evaluated as the clients perceive them to be—not as the clients think they are *supposed* to be. An example I usually give the group is a needs circle done by an alcoholic. It shows clearly the lack of meaningful relationships and depicts the only need-fulfilling activity as drinking.

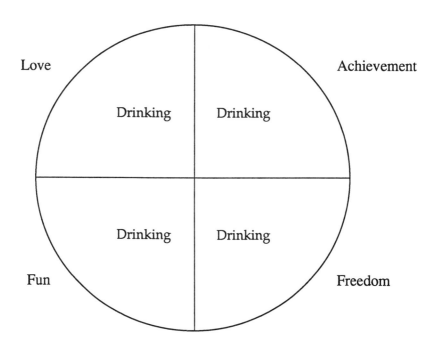

Once we have evaluated the behavior of drinking and how that has affected a person's needs (by not filling them), we move on to other so-called "problem" behaviors. The group members evaluate their own past behaviors quite readily. Janet, who has an eating disorder, draws a needs circle very similar to the drinker's, with food replacing alcohol in every quadrant. Laurel, the co-dependent client, completes her circle with certain controlling actions, such as complying with her abusive spouse. With the idea that their behaviors do not have to make "sense" to anyone, including themselves, the groups seem to enjoy the process of examining in detail what needs they are trying to meet.

Next, we take a look at how we are getting our needs met in our relationships. With so many unsuccessful attempts at getting their needs met with activities such as drinking or binge-eating, they are open to the idea that they are probably not getting their needs met through their relationships either.

Now we draw an individual needs circle for each group member in much the same way that we drew the relationship diagrams previously. One at a time, the group members evaluate their lives and relationships according to how various people and activities have been meeting their needs. There are a couple things to watch out for while the clients are doing these evaluations. Quite often they will emerge with a needs circle that is based on appearances. If a client has a relationship with someone, but that relationship is not helping the client to meet any of his needs, then the client should not include that person on the chart. Laurel, for instance, is tempted to put her alcoholic spouse in as helping to meet her need for love, but she does not persist when asked to evaluate whether the spouse is *really* meeting that need. When Laurel completed her needs circle, it looked like this:

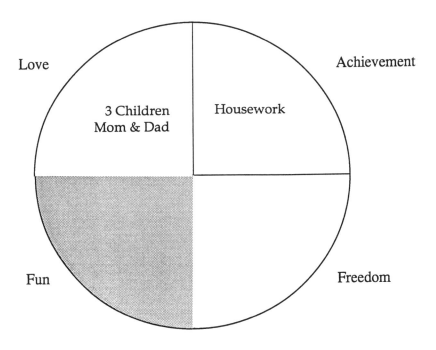

It is important that the clients evaluate what is actually going on in their lives, not how they would like us or themselves to see things. This is once again a time when counseling skills are brought to bear. If the client persists, then it is, after all, the client's evaluation. Besides, they often have more than one opportunity to make this evaluation, so they may see things differently the next time.

Sometimes situations need to be clarified by breaking them down into people and activities. For instance, clients often report that they derive considerable enjoyment from their job or school. When queried, it may turn out that they enjoy the people, but not the activity, in which case they should include only their co-workers or schoolmates as being need-fulfilling in their needs circle. Or sometimes it is the other way around; Marge loves doing her job, but cannot stand her co-workers. In this case, the job is included in the appropriate places of her needs circle, but the co-workers are not included at all.

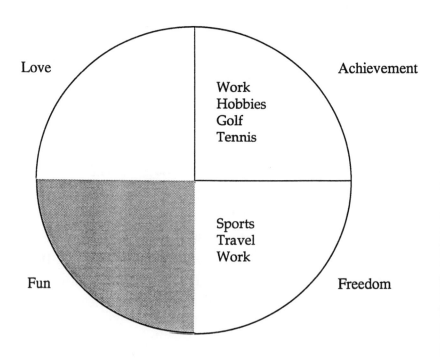

Commonly, clients arrive at the conclusion that one or more of their needs are not being met at all. Robert, the teenager, sees relationships with his friends as meeting both his need for belonging and for freedom. His mother, girlfriend, and car are also included in his circle, but he indicates nothing that is meeting his need for achievement.

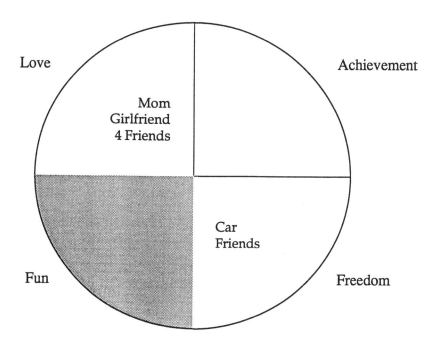

Anita's circle is almost empty. A perpetual student, Anita has already received several degrees in different fields, and she is currently in pursuit of yet another. She sees school as meeting her need for achievement, but can think of no relationships with classmates, professors, or anyone else, as need-fulfilling. Anita's circle looks like this:

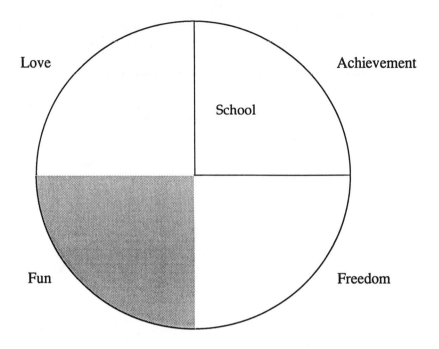

While Albert's needs circle (below) appears balanced in that there are no empty quadrants, he has no alternatives for satisfying his needs. He often finds himself in situations where he is unable to meet his needs.

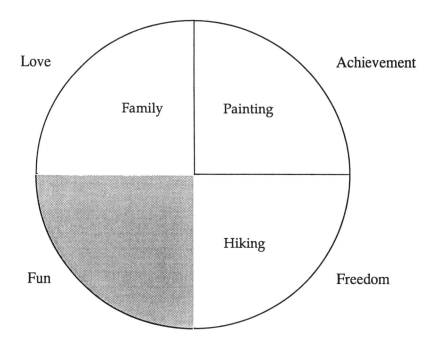

We go through this exercise one person at a time, giving everyone an equal chance to evaluate. The repetition reiterates that when our needs are not being met, we must do something to try to meet our needs! To connect the information I ask each client as we go around the room, "What do you think you have been doing to get your needs met?" Again, we talk of behavior as an attempt at the time to meet a need, even though it does not make sense to the person doing it. An example of this is George, the alcoholic, who returns to drinking in spite of his life falling apart. When we go through this needs analysis in group, everyone evaluates George's drinking from the perspective of, "Well, he has to do something, doesn't he?"

Next come the crucial questions. "Have these activities been getting you what you want? How has it been working out? What do you think you could start doing instead?" Most often, I get the old blank stares again. Few have any idea of what to do that is different. Make no mistake, they are aware of options, but these options do not yet seem viable to them. Therefore, we redo the needs circles to represent what the client perceives would be their quality world of relationships. Again, all are included so that everyone has some input. A quality world circle of need-fulfilling relationships for Laurel looks like this:

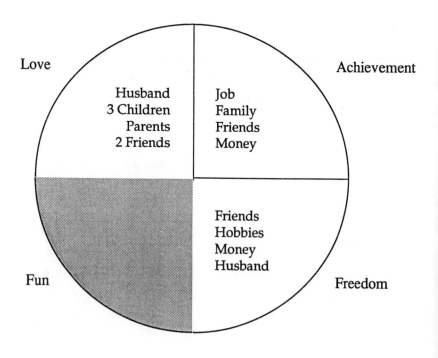

At this stage we compare the value of someone continuously trying to get what they think they want versus the value of someone trying to learn to meet their needs. It is simpler to learn to meet four or five needs than it is to continue trying to obtain the thousands of wants that attract our attention daily. I carefully point out that although it is simpler, it is not necessarily any easier. From personal experience I know that it will become easier, but it may not start out that way.

We then discuss specific behaviors that the individuals can use to help get their own needs met, to make their current needs circle match their quality world needs circle. Robert, for example, wants to start getting some of his love and belonging needs met at home with both his parents. Up to this point he has largely blamed his father for the breakdown in their relationship. Now he sees that if he wants his father to meet his need for love and belonging he must take some of the responsibility himself. One way that he thinks he can do this is to start telling the truth instead of lies. We discuss in the group what "telling the truth" would look like. The group decides that telling the truth one hundred percent of the time now and forever will probably not work as a plan for Robert—it is too big a change for him to make so suddenly. An alternate suggestion, telling one or two truths, is not acceptable either. That would be too few. Robert settles on telling twenty-two truths before the group meets again.

The last part of this session is spent on the general things that can be done to help get the clients' needs met in their relationships—where to go to socialize, to get the support they are looking for, what that support would look like, etc. As usual the group ends on this positive note, focusing not on the failures but on solutions to their challenges. The needs circle exercise gives individuals in the group a common-sense idea about why they are or are not comfortable with the various situations in their lives. Afterwards, they continue to evaluate their relationships and situations on a "needs met" basis.

SOLUTIONS
Stage Eight

KEY QUESTIONS
Are you interested in finding something else to do that will get you what you really want?
Is it easily attainable?
Is it an action that is reportable?
Is it something you want to do?
Will you benefit by doing it once?
If you keep doing it, will it meet your needs?

ACTIVITIES
Evaluating fantasies for evidence of unmet needs
Planning win/win solutions

Throughout the Solution Group process the clients have been working on solutions. Whether speaking of feeling better, thinking differently, or doing different things, the clients have been seeking new choices or alternatives to unwanted behaviors. At times, the solutions seem repetitive, but as the group progresses, the variety and effectiveness of the solutions increase. Arriving at solutions each day and going home with something the client can actually do is fundamental to the Solution Group process. Clients often start out thinking that changing their lives is next to impossible—haven't they tried it many times before, without success? The daily solutions, carefully designed to provide immediate results, help convince them they can do it! Clients also come into the group looking for suggestions for "fixing" their lives. Most of the time they expect me to give them the answers that will change their lives. One of the counselor's most important chores is convincing the clients that they never will be told what to do.

In the beginning of the discussion we talk about the value of trying to change old behaviors. I remind them of the Christmas tree analogy presented earlier in the discussion of actions. It is important for the clients to understand that when we are talking about solutions, we are talking of starting new behaviors, not changing or "shining up" old behaviors. The new behaviors are not designed to help the client get rid of something, but should help the client get something that he or she needs, or really wants.

It may appear that searching for new behaviors to meet a client's needs is a process of trial and error. After the self-evaluations have been done by the group, the clients are well aware of what they have been feeling, thinking, and doing that is not effective, but how do they decide what new behaviors can be effectively substituted for the old? There is a sort of system to direct clients to the new behaviors that will have a high likelihood of success. In the early stages of the group process, the counselor must subtly guide the clients to appropriate interim solutions, but at this stage the group is ready to discuss the solution-making process in detail.

Successful solutions are what I call "win/win solutions." A win/win solution meets a client's needs, not necessarily their tangible wants. When the client can answer "Yes" to the following questions about a proposed solution, then they have found a win/win solution.

1) Is it easily attainable?
2) Is it an action (i.e., not a thought or feeling)?
3) Is it something you want to do?
4) Will you benefit by doing it once?
5) If you keep doing it, will it meet your needs?

To enhance the chances for initial success, a time limit should be set for attempting or accomplishing the new activity, and the person should report what happens, thereby marking their own success by telling someone else.

To get the group on the track of devising win/win solutions, we review the five basic needs— L.A.F.F.S.—and talk of all the unwanted behaviors the group listed in previous sessions and how they are really attempts by the client to meet their needs. While it may not make sense for George to keep on drinking or Laurel to keep on making excuses for her abusive husband, these behaviors represent the best these clients could do at the time. The important question for George and Laurel, and all other clients, is, "Are you interested in finding something else to do that will get you what you really want?"

Although we have talked about the clients' wants and needs in previous sessions, the clients at this stage may still not have a clear idea of how their wants and needs are related. Since the best solutions meet both a client's needs and wants, the clients must clarify their personal interpretations of these before they start planning solutions. For identifying their needs, or establishing the very personal nature of the needs, I ask the group members to go off somewhere by themselves and write down on a piece of paper a fantasy about something they would like to be doing, somewhere they would like to be, something they would like to have. Whatever they have for a fantasy is okay. There is no need for it to be remotely possible or attainable. If they would like to raise horses and potatoes on Hawaii, that's great. Then, we gather back in the group and as each person reads his or her fantasy the group evaluates the needs that the fantasy reveals. The rationale for this exercise is that if a need is already being met, the client will have no desire to fantasize about a time when it will be met.

To give them an example, I describe a fantasy of my own. When I first did this exercise during my reality therapy training, my fantasy was to be at a lake cottage in northern Saskatchewan. In my fantasy, I saw myself sitting on a dock, feet swinging in the water, the sun coming up, and loons out on the water singing. The greatest unmet need represented by my fantasy, I decided, was a need for freedom.

Janet says she dreams of living on the coast, with no responsibilities, where she can walk on the beach every day and write for a living. Janet had come into the group claiming to be unloved, unwanted, and lonely—thinking her greatest need was for love and belonging. The fantasy exercise reveals to her a need to feel free. In Ted's fantasy we recognize the need for power. He envisions himself building tall skyscrapers in large cities which will live long after him. Anita sees herself at home gathered in front of a cozy fireplace with three children and a dog, then walking in the woods holding hands with someone she really loves. "We would know everything about each other and understand each other completely." The group understands that Anita's greatest need is for love and belonging.

After everyone has done the fantasy exercise, we use the needs revealed by the fantasies as a starting point for finding win/win solutions. The clients are quite certain they will never realize their fantasies, but I tell them they can at least do something to help to meet the needs that their fantasies have revealed. I present to them the concept of the win/win solution, telling them that the challenge is to find something to do that can lead to meeting their needs or getting something they want, but no matter what the result, just doing the activity will be good for them. Again, I use myself as an example.

At one time the place where I worked forbade smoking by staff. Although I had tried many times to quit, I was a smoker. I hated sneaking cigarettes in the basement when the weather was too ugly to go outside—and there are lots of ugly days in the winters of Saskatchewan. I felt trapped. In search of a solution, I made a win/win decision to start swimming at the YMCA. Swimming was something I liked to do, and it could possibly get me what I wanted to quit smoking. There was no way to lose; the worst that could happen was that I would continue to smoke. I joined the YMCA and began to swim laps. Within two weeks I realized I had to choose between swimming and smoking—I could not do both. I chose swimming and haven't had one puff since.

How can clients find win/win solutions on a daily basis for the huge challenges that they face? An essential guideline is to keep all solutions at a level of manageability. Clients have a tendency to want to do too much too fast. They want to tackle the whole mountain and move it, today! It does the client a great disservice to encourage choices that are not likely to succeed. Usually, grandiose ideas can be shaped into activities that are manageable.

Janet, for instance, says she wants to leave home and get out on her own. She has become empowered during this group process. She cannot, however, really see herself doing this. She has tried before and not succeeded. As we talk further, she states that she always tried to leave without any support. So the question becomes whether she feels she can get what she wants if she starts to get the necessary support around her. Then later she can review her options. We decide that Janet may be able to find the support she is looking for if she develops contacts in the community. This way she will not have to rely on her home situation to get all her needs met. She says that she used to tutor students in reading and enjoyed it very much. She misses doing it. Janet commits to inquiring about the local literacy group's volunteer tutoring program and will report back to the group tomorrow. She can't lose. Even if she never moves out on her own, she will have become involved in an activity that meets her needs for belonging, achievement, freedom, and fun. The idea of increasing community contacts, gathering support, and suspending the final decision about whether or not to leave home is an effective, win/win solution for Janet.

Ted's case is different. Not viewing himself as a drug addict, Ted expresses the desire to "smoke a little pot occasionally—just when I'm with my friends, you know." Every time he gets involved with drugs, though, he ends up in trouble, most often in jail. His most recent escapades landed him in the group via a parole order. When Ted expresses his desire to be a social marijuana smoker, I say, "Go ahead!"

He is shocked. "I thought your job was to get me to quit doing drugs all together!"

I give him my regrets and ask him if that would work anyway. He agrees that neither I nor anyone else can get him to quit unless he wants to. Now we agree on one thing—it is Ted's job to look after his drug use. My giving him permission to go ahead and do what he wants is an open door. I don't hold the power to tell anyone what to do, but I do ask lots of questions.

"Ted, before you decide to smoke dope with your friends, I would like to ask you a couple of questions. Number one, what happens to you when you do drugs? And two, does it get you what you want?"

Sometimes the truth makes a reluctant appearance, but it will come. With Ted, it comes easily. I ask him what is the likelihood he will have the same results the next time he uses marijuana. After his evaluation I once again stress that he can do whatever he wants, but he might want to keep the consequences in mind when deciding. If he is interested in other choices or solutions, we can look for some. In Ted's case, it turns out that he wants to do something to meet his need for love and belonging. Because he has already made some contacts with a local halfway house, which he views positively, it is relatively simple for him to come up with a win/win solution. Ted decides to renew his acquaintances there by making a phone call that evening to the resident director. He will report back to the group the next day. Ted, too, has found a win/win solution that is at a manageable level.

Laurel, like many abused clients, came to the group looking for someone to tell her how to get away from her abusive situation or how to change the behavior of her abusive husband. Through the Solution Group process, Laurel has begun to see that she has legitimate needs and that her "powerlessness" is the root of her problems. Furthermore, she has begun to realize that there is nothing she can do to change her husband's behavior; she can only change her own. She thinks that perhaps she should move out of the house, but quickly decides that this would be impossible for her to do. She believes her husband really cares for her, she knows of no place to go, and she has no means of supporting herself and her children. Out of the group discussion, however, comes a win/win solution. She decides that even if she cannot move out of the house, when her husband starts to become abusive she can tell him she isn't going to tolerate it any longer and immediately leave the room. I urge Laurel to think of a second solution as well. It is important that she have something she can do that is

totally independent of the abusive person, something outside the abusive situation. Because she
always enjoyed and got good grades in her art
classes at school and says she admires the independ-
ence and eccentricities of "artsy" people, she decides
she will sign up to take an art class. She reports to
the group that the plans work! Refusing to tolerate
any abuse removes her from potentially abusive
situations before they can escalate, and standing up
to her husband in this way enhances her feeling of
power and achievement. The first art class she
attended was fun and she says the other people are
very "interesting"; she's looking forward to getting
to know them better. Laurel is finding out for herself
that devising successful win/win solutions is, itself,
an empowering process.

Helping Albert find a win/win solution is not
too difficult because despite his extreme loneliness,
which is related to his need for love and belonging,
he has many family members (real and honorary),
some of whom live in the same city. Re-establishing
a relationship with just one person will be a start.
When I ask Albert how he could go about doing this,
he says, "I suppose I could go visit my aunt. She
doesn't live too far away and I haven't seen her in a
while." Knowing that alcoholism and extreme
poverty are frequent problems for native Americans
living in urban settings, I check that the results of
Albert's visit are likely to be beneficial. "Is she living
the way you want to live?" Albert answers, "Sort of.
She's clean, and sober, and she's been good to me

before." That sounds good enough to me. "So when are you going to see her?" I ask. "Tonight, I guess," says Albert. "I'll tell you about it tomorrow."

Remember that this type of discussion is far from being a tearing-down process. All the discussions are carried out in a respectful manner and are solution-oriented. Furthermore, ideas for the solutions come from the clients themselves and are crafted with the help of the leader and the group to meet the client's needs, interests, and situation. Whether the solutions are for large challenges or small, they deserve respectful attention. The solutions discussed here as examples may not seem especially substantial in proportion to the enormity of the clients' problems, but they are very effective when measured against the potential for success. You have to start somewhere—you can't climb a mountain until you have gone through the foothills. The clients will continue to progress as they experience success and make further choices. Ultimate success in meeting their needs and getting what they really want is possible only when each step forward is manageable and satisfies the criteria of a win/win solution.

GOOD-BYES AND FOLLOW-UP
Stage Nine

KEY QUESTION
What are one or two positive qualities you have noticed about each person in the group?

ACTIVITY
Telling each person, in turn, the nice things everyone has noticed

In keeping with the spirit of the Solution Group process, the good-byes send everyone off on a positive note. The group just spends time together saying what they like about each other. In the good-bye activity every person in the group tells one or two nice things they have noticed about each of the other group members since they met them. There is no "helpful feedback," no advice, nothing like "I think you need to...," or "You should...," or even "When you get it together...." In short, no comments are made that could be construed as critical. The comments should be spoken aloud, because written comments tend to be repetitive and sound insincere. It's best if the time for this activity is not limited. Everyone in the group needs to have their moment as the center of attention while everyone else, in turn, says something nice about them. I advise everyone ahead of time that this session will take "as long as it takes." We usually run longer than planned, but no one minds. The clients enjoy saying and hearing the sincere compliments that are given and received about themselves and everyone else.

Let me give some examples of comments people make to their fellow group members. Comments offered to Charles include, "I like your honesty...your humor...the way you are willing to make changes...the way you are devoted to your kids." The group says to Janet, "I like your determination...your honesty...your warmth...how smart you are...how eager you are to learn." To Laurel they say, "I like the way you have accepted your new role in your life...how you have already gone out and tried what you have learned...the way you accept others...the friendly way you welcomed me into the group." An interesting sidelight of these good-byes is that the compliments usually start out being quite short and relatively non-specific. As the activity gets going and everyone gets involved, the compliments get longer, more complex, and more innovative! Even clients as reticent as Albert have no trouble participating and being included in this activity. The sorts of things Albert hears about himself are, "I like your smile...your courage and determination...your patience...that you are a wonderful, 'safe' person to be around." The nice things Albert says to others include, "I like your humor...the way you ask questions...your honesty...the way you accept people."

When I first started the Solution Group process, I did not include myself in this good-bye activity, I guess because I viewed the group as being for the benefit of the clients and felt, in a sense, that I was apart from the group. When I sat in on a group run by someone else, however, I found it very rewarding to have the group leader included in this good-bye activity as well. Now I allow the individuals in the group to give me their comments if they wish, and they always choose to do so. By having this chance to say good-bye to me, they are helped to feel that they are ready to move on in life.

All in all, it takes a minimum of 24-30 hours to get through all nine stages of the Solution Group. The time can be spread out, however, in various formats. Sometimes I have done two-hour sessions on consecutive evenings for two weeks. It is possible to hold the group sessions once a week for two or three months, but I have found this arrangement less effective than more concentrated programs. Recently I have been conducting Solution Groups as an intensive process, completing all the stages and activities within a four-day period, often during a long weekend starting Thursday evening and meeting all day on Friday, Saturday and Sunday. With this format, one stage follows another directly, and the clients must absorb ideas and information rapidly. Even though every endeavor is made to ensure that every client is "on board" at every stage, the group members often feel they need more time to reflect on the process and the impact it can have on their lives. In response to many requests, the Solution Group process now includes a series of eight 2-hour follow-up sessions at weekly intervals following completion of the initial concentrated program. Each session is a brief recap of the essential questions and activities of the Solution Group stages. We make a point of devising new win/win solutions for each participant at the end of each session.

OVERVIEW

Having just completed an initial exposure to the process, you, the reader, may appreciate a brief recap of the Solution Group stages.

The process begins with introductions to acquaint the group members with each other and with the process. The Solution Group proves to be different from what most people have experienced or expected. They do not spend their time going into grand confessions, nor do they have to explain their various behaviors. Clients do not have to tell the group about their awful pains, their awful thoughts,

119

or the awful things that they have done. Some of this information will surface, incidentally, but it is not the main focus of the introductions, nor of the process as a whole. In this first stage, we find out some of what the clients want to be doing, and eventually, what they have really been wanting in their lives. And the clients learn that what they want is what this group is all about. They are promised a safe environment. There will be no criticism. They will not be told what to do. They will make their own decisions. Clients have told me that the benefits of the Solution Group process start with the introductions.

In the second stage, the clients look at their feelings, specifically those that they have not liked. Again, there is no element of confession here, and the various feelings discussed are not necessarily the ones the clients are having today. Each member of the group is asked to add to a list at least one feeling that they have had, at any time in their lives, that they did not like. When the list is complete they are asked to evaluate how these feelings have been working for them, as well as the overall amount of time and energy that they have put into these feelings. And we discuss the "root of it all"—fear. We discuss the nature of fear, how it affects all of our lives, and how it can lead to a host of other bad feelings, most of which will be on the list compiled by the group. The idea is discussed that fear itself is not such a terrible thing; the ability to respond to a threat is really a desirable behavior. Whenever we feel threatened, when we perceive an unmet need, we must behave in some manner to get what we want; we must try some behavior to meet our needs. Next we list the feelings the clients would like to be having, and we talk about some strategies for feeling better.

In the third stage, the focus is on the clients' thoughts, particularly their thoughts about themselves and how these may be related to their feelings. A brief exercise introduces them to the idea that thoughts can produce feelings and that it is not possible simply to *stop* thinking something or to *stop* feeling something—one must *start* thinking or feeling something else. As we did with feelings they didn't like having, we compile a list of thoughts about themselves that they do not like and ask, if that is what they are thinking, how would they expect to feel? This is followed by a discussion of what they would be thinking if they were happy, and what they can do to start thinking that way.

In the fourth stage, we concentrate on actions, or things they are doing. All the clients have done many things they are not proud of, things they would prefer not to be doing. As before, we make a list, this time of the unwanted actions. The clients always wonder why they do all these things, many of which don't seem to make any sense. In providing a rationale, I explain the control theory/reality therapy concept of the five basic needs—Love, Achievement, Freedom, Fun, and Survival—and how whenever one of our needs is not being met, we must do something to try to meet that need. Whenever a need is unmet or threatened, a person behaves in some manner that is an attempt to get something that he or she wants to meet that need. The major question is, how effectively do certain behaviors meet their needs? Once again the group compiles the companion list—the things the clients want to be doing, and we talk about what the clients would be thinking and feeling if they were doing those things.

In the fifth stage we examine how changes in our physiology or health represent another component of behavior in the sense that they may be attempts to meet thwarted needs. Physiology is the final element of total behavior that the group focuses on. Once each of the four components of behavior have been discussed, total behavior is evaluated for each client using Dr. Glasser's "Control Car" model. The important concept is that all the components of total behavior affect each other, but "thinking" and "doing" dominate "feeling" and "physiology." We imagine what the ideal or quality "car" would look like and start to discuss specific behaviors the group members can use to start getting them what they want. By the end of the fifth stage, the clients have come up with a full list of how they would like to be feeling emotionally, thinking, acting, and feeling health-wise. The discussion turns to what these things that they have been wanting would look like. This gets their minds off all the terrible "stuff" that they have been doing all of their lives. It gets them talking about their "wants" and not their "faults." The group members spend a great deal of time and energy developing their mental pictures of what their various wants would look like.

Having evaluated and discussed all the elements of total behavior, the clients move in the sixth stage to evaluating how their various behaviors have affected their personal relationships. They evaluate the effect their own behaviors have had not only on people around them, but also on themselves and their own best interests. They consider what their own "best interests" would be.

In the seventh stage, they chart on a needs circle how their needs for love or belonging, achievement or power, freedom, and fun are being met by their relationships and activities. In this stage they evaluate their relationships based on which needs they are meeting in a meaningful way, and eventually the clients start to evaluate how they would like to better meet their needs in the future. Strategies are discussed for how to accomplish this.

In the eighth stage we discuss strategies for how to begin the process of actually doing something to meet the clients' needs. We begin with the exercise where they write out their fantasies. From this exercise, which most clients find is fun to do, we discover one or two unmet needs for each client. From identifying unmet needs, we move on to things the clients can do to meet these needs. I acquaint them with the idea of win/win solutions and how to apply them. Briefly, a win/win solution is easy to accomplish, is an action that is reportable, and is something that the client wants to do. Furthermore, if the client does it only once, it will be beneficial, and if they keep it up, it will help them meet their need. The group leader's job is to help the clients shape their ideas into manageable, win/win solutions so that the clients will better meet their needs and, ultimately, get what they really want.

The positive focus and congenial atmosphere of the Solution Group is clearly demonstrated when the leader and group members exchange pleasant thoughts about each other in the good-bye session. Now that the group is disbanding, what has been accomplished? The clients have gained some new insights into their old behaviors. They have begun to realize that they are not weak people, but rather, they are strong people, trying things all the time to right the "wrongs" in their lives. They realize that they may have to start changing what they do, not who they are. They have redirected blame toward self-evaluation and have begun perfecting self-evaluation skills. They have gained experience and achieved success in devising win/win solutions for some of their problems. They will not have solved all their problems, but they will have started an on-going process of self-evaluation, based on the question "How is that working out for you?" They have started the process of changing their behavior so they are more likely to get what they really want and need in the long run.

APPENDIX

IF YOU WANT TO LEAD A SOLUTION GROUP...
The philosophical framework and necessary counseling skills for Solution Group leaders are best developed by training in reality therapy and control theory through the certification process of the Institute for Reality Therapy 7301 Medical Center Drive, Suite 104, Canoga Park, CA 91307. Further training specifically for leaders of Solution Groups is provided by Quality Group Counseling, Inc. Call 1-800-667-3555 for further information.

I encourage you to adopt and adapt the strategies and activities I have described in this book, but remember, please, that the name "The Solution Group" is a registered trade-mark of Quality Group Counseling, Inc. (2320 Cornwall Street, Regina, Saskatchewan, Canada S4P2L3). Any use of the trade-mark is strictly prohibited without the written permission of the owner.

ADDITIONAL READING

Sources for further information about reality therapy and control theory include:

Boffey, Barnes. *Reinventing Yourself.* Chapel Hill, NC: New View Publications, 1993.

Glasser, William. *Reality Therapy.* New York: HarperCollins, 1969.

Glasser, William. *Control Theory.* New York: HarperCollins, 1984.

Glasser, Naomi. *Control Theory in the Practice of Reality Therapy.* New York: HarperCollins, 1989.

Good, Perry. *In Pursuit of Happiness.* Chapel Hill, NC: New View Publications, 1987.

Wubbolding, Robert. *Understanding Reality Therapy.* New York: HarperCollins, 1991.

Wubbolding, Robert. *Using Reality Therapy.* New York: HarperCollins, 1988.